POWER FAILURE

A nurse's story

Terri Arthur, RN

Other books by Terri Arthur

Fatal Decision: Edith Cavell WWI Nurse, 2nd edition.

*Fatal Destiny: Edith Cavell WWI Nurse,
    British edition.*

*Audio CD's and MP3's, of Fatal Destiny: Edith Cavell
WW1 Nurse read by British actress Laura Jane
    Waitling*

*Nurse Hero: Edith Cavell, children's edition
    with study guide*

POWER FAILURE

A nurse's story

Terri Arthur, RN

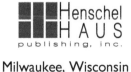

Milwaukee, Wisconsin

Published by
HenschelHAUS Publishing, Inc.
Milwaukee, Wisconsin
www.henschelHAUSbooks.com

ISBN (KDP paperback): 979877321-762-6
ISBN (LSI paperback): 978159598-873-7
ISBN: (hardcover, special edition): 978159598-874-4
E-ISBN: 978159598-866-9
LCCN: 2021945373

Printed in the United States of America

*They whispered to her, "You cannot
withstand the storm."
She whispered back, "I am the storm."*
~Jake Remington

*Dedicated to my nursing colleagues
who weather the storm
every day they go to work.*

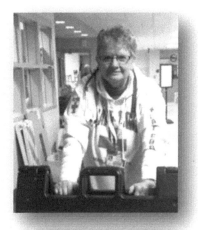

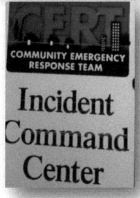

TABLE OF CONTENTS

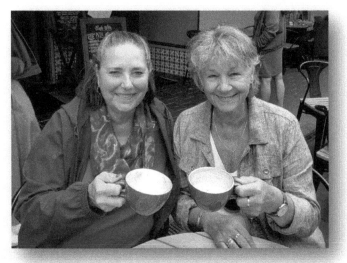

Kira Henschel (L), publisher and Linda Callaghan (R) cover designer, enjoying a cuppa together in New Zealand where Linda lives.

ACKNOWLEDGEMENTS

Evelyn Bain, RN, who encouraged the writing of this book, listened to my ideas—good and bad—read my manuscript draft, and made helpful suggestions.

Cathy Dicker, RN, my marketing manager, who read through my manuscript and offered excellent advice on content and line editing.

Vicky Wilson-Schwartz, Ph.D., my premier editor, who has the patience of Job, the vision of Solomon, and the ability to understand what I meant to say.

Linda Callaghan, my award-winning cover designer from New Zealand, who patiently worked with me to create the cover of this book.

Kira Henschel, my publisher, who has made all of my books possible.

AUTHOR'S NOTE

My story starts with one word: *bombogenesis*. It was the description given to the combined hurricane and blizzard named "Nemo" that struck the East Coast on February 8, 2013. The name Nemo had nothing to do with the colorful, cute, cuddly Disney fish who sadly lost his way in the vast ocean. This storm hit the East Coast with a fierceness that other storms will be compared to for decades.

I was reluctant to write about my experience during this storm, which was rated as one of the worst five storms in this century. I pondered that I might have failed in some way. Now, eight years later, it still haunts me. I continue to wonder what else I could have done.

NEW ENGLAND'S NEWSPAPER OF THE YEAR

CAPE COD TIMES

capecodONLINE.com

The Cape and Islands' Daily Newspaper

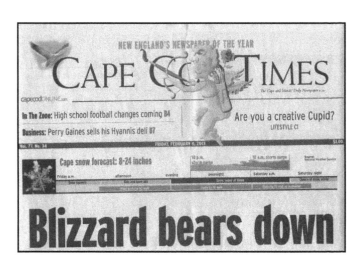

In The Zone: High school football changes coming B4

Business: Perry Gaines sells his Hyannis deli B7

Are you a creative Cupid?
LIFESTYLE C1

Vol. 77, No. 34   FRIDAY, FEBRUARY 8, 2013 $1.00

Cape snow forecast: 8-24 inches

Friday a.m.	afternoon	evening	overnight	Saturday a.m.	Saturday night

10 p.m. storm surge

10 a.m. storm surge

Source: National Weather Service

Blizzard bears down

Chapter 1

OPENING UP THE MEDICAL CLINIC

Monday, February 8, 2013

My morning began as so many had before until my eyes locked onto the *Cape Cod Times* headlines, and then darted down to the story.

> *Much of Cape Cod is shutting down in anticipation of a blizzard that is forecast to bring high winds and heavy snow to the region this weekend. Area safety officials held a conference call Thursday afternoon to discuss storm preparation plans.*

I skipped down the article.

> *Cape Cod could get anywhere from 3 to 5 feet of snow, maybe more and wind gusts up to 80mph. Travel will be severely impeded. Cape Air has canceled all flights*

to the New England states and New York. The Martha's Vineyard and Nantucket Steamship Authority is canceling ferry service until Sunday. Bus services to Boston has been stopped.

Shelters will be open when the storm starts.

I stared at the satellite photo in disbelief. The entire East Coast from Virginia to Nova Scotia was going to be hit.

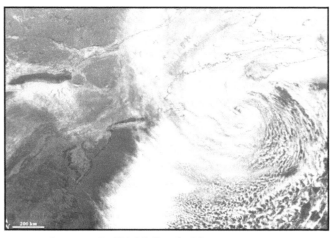

Image via NASA Earth Observatory
Cape Cod Times February 8, 2013

Beneath the picture I read:

> *Atmospheric blend for a behemoth storm is expected to move slowly, creating 36 hours of rapid snowfall. The fierce nor'easter that will be walloping New England tonight is a formation of two converging storms that is merging, causing a rapidly strengthening storm known in weather jargon as a "meteorological bomb" or "bombogenesis."*

"Bombogeneis." I needed to say the unfamiliar word out loud to believe it existed. I still didn't quite understand it. I searched the rest of the article for some mistake in the prediction. Maybe the storm will blow out to sea or the barometric pressure won't drop as fast or the winds will shift or...

The phone rang.

"Have you heard the weather prediction?"

I instantly recognized the voice of Alice Kent-Levinson, Chief Nurse of the local Red Cross Chapter. Her accent still carried the remnants of New York City, where she once lived. My hand tightened around the phone because I knew what was coming next.

"We need you to open up the health service at the Shelton shelter, and we need you to do it as soon as possible before the snow starts. Governor Patrick is ordering all vehicles be banned from public roads after 4:00pm today. Anyone who violates this order will be penalized with a year in jail or a $500 fine, except, of course, for emergency vehicles or workers. Pack up to be prepared to stay at the shelter for at least two days, possibly three. Are you okay with this?"

"I've never stayed at a shelter that long, but I'll be okay." I modulated my voice to sound casual. "No problem." I lied. "I'll be there in about an hour."

I was about to hang up when she added, "One more thing. I'll be off-duty tonight so I can be awake to take calls in the morning, when it will be busy. Betty will be taking the night shift. You have her number?"

"I'm sure I do." (Somewhere in my scrambled, dog-eared, crossed-out, falling-apart address book.)

I had opened up the medical clinic in these shelters before but never alone and never for three days. There was always a nurse assigned to work with me. I tried to sound confident, but I felt my voice falter a bit. "Who, ah, who will be working with me?"

I heard a hesitation in her voice. "I...I'm not sure. They are opening up four of the six shelters on the Cape, and all of my nurses have already been assigned." Her voice trailed off and then picked up.

"I'll call the Medical Corps to see if they can send us someone, but as you are the Red Cross nurse, you will be in charge. We have no time to waste. This storm will bring down power lines. That means people without electricity will be crowding into the shelters. Be prepared for a busy few days. They said it will be one of the worst five storms we've had in a century. It's going to be the storm every-one will be talking about for years to come."

I hauled out my canvas boat bag and filled it with personal items, a stethoscope, a flash-light, and a change of clothes. I also knew from past experiences that the food at these shelters was never in line for the James Beard

Restaurant Award, so I packed two bananas, two instant oatmeal containers, a package of chocolate chip cookies, and peanut butter crackers.

My partner, Elaine, whose personality matches her flaming red hair, watched the weather predictions on a Boston TV station then walked into the kitchen and saw me packing the cookies. "Oh no, tell me that doesn't mean what I think it means. You aren't going to do the shelter again, are you?"

"Elaine, I have to go. It's my job as a Red Cross nurse. I volunteered to do this."

"There are a hundred other nurses on the Cape. Let them be the heroes."

"Actually, there are thousands of other nurses on the Cape, but only a half dozen of them are trained by the Red Cross to run the medical services in the shelters. I'm one of them."

"There's only six of them with good reason. Not many nurses are willing to take on this responsibility. It's dangerous and you are on your own with little to no medical support. Why put yourself through this?" Elaine said.

"Someone has to do it. It might as well be the nurse with forty years of critical care nursing, don't you think?"

Her emerald eyes narrowed. "I think, Miss Florence Nightingale, that I will be worrying about you the entire time you are away. Promise to call me when you get there and every few hours."

"I will. Don't worry. I've done this three times before and it's always worked out. Actually, I like the challenge. It's kind of fun."

"Only you would think it's 'kind of fun' to be stuck in some God-forsaken shelter in the middle of a blizzard or a hurricane, and in this case it's frickin' both, with a bunch of sick people."

I walked over, put my arms around her, and pulled her close to me. The hair on top of her head brushed against my chin. "Don't worry, sweetheart. I'm with a bunch of other people as crazy as I am."

"And that's supposed to make me feel better?"

I called my sister, Gail, who lives across the street from us. "Hey, kiddo. Just to let

7

you know that I'm heading out for the Red Cross shelter in Shelton."

"Oh no. Why do you have to do this? I hate it when you leave home to work in the shelters. I always worry about you."

I loved my sister. She is ten years younger than me. While growing up, I was her "other Mom" while my mother worked. Gail was always kind and compassionate, the kind of person who always finds the bird with the broken wing and takes it in.

"So let me get this right," I said. "This is coming from the only white woman who worked in the Bronx for years as a Salvation Army officer. I remember visiting you and seeing bullet holes in the door to the building where you lived. Your neighborhood seemed like a war zone. Every building around you looked like you lived in Beirut. The rats were the size of cats and ate through your walls.

"I remember you getting calls to do a funeral service for someone they found buried in a cement wall when the building fell apart. And you're worried about how safe I'll be in a high school filled with dedicated people all working to provide safety to people who have nowhere else to go?"

"You were born a rescuer," Gail said.

"So were you. It must be genetic."

"Please promise to call me every couple of hours and tell me you are okay."

"I promise, but promise me you'll check in on Elaine. She hasn't been through one of our Cape storms. She gets very upset when I work the shelters, and will be especially worried in a storm this massive. She is used to roads being cleared more quickly and had fewer problems with losing electricity when she lived in her apartment in Boston."

"Of course I'll keep an eye out for her. She can always stay with me if she wants to."

"Thanks for offering. Please tell her that but don't be disappointed if she refuses."

Elaine slung my boat bag over her shoulder, broadened from years of swimming and diving. She walked with me to the car and heaved the bag into the backseat. She put her face close to mine to give me her usual good-bye warnings "Wear your seatbelt. Drive carefully. Come home safely to me."

As I drove to the high school shelter, I noticed the brightness of the skies fade away to an army of dark gunmetal-gray clouds marching along the horizon. The air was swollen with the promise of snow and seemed hemmed in by a draining and impending gloom.

Along the way, I saw people moving their cars into garages or in open areas away from trees. A few were nailing boards across their picture windows. I passed a Stop-and-Shop. The parking lot was jammed with cars. People rushed from the store pushing carriages filled

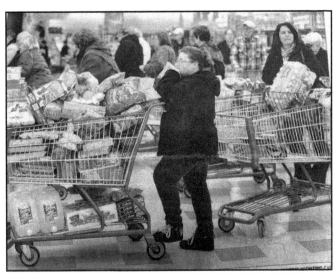

Cape Cod Times, February 8, 2013

with bottles of water and toilet paper. I passed a gas station. The line of cars spilled out into the street and lined up along the curb.

Two blocks from the high school, I suddenly stopped. The road was blocked with a wooden barricade on two sawhorses. A sign with large red letters hung in the middle. "DO NOT PASS," it read. I looked for someone monitoring the blocked road who could give out directions for a detour, but found no one. I backed out and attempted to take my own detour but I was met with yet another blockade.

"How in the hell were people supposed to reach the shelter if even the staff can't even get there?" I wondered. "Enough," I said out loud. I got out of the car, moved the wooden barrier aside, drove through, and put it back in place.

I found a parking place easily enough and walked past an ambulance that was parked in front of the entrance. I could feel the temperature of the wind become colder on my cheeks. Two EMTs hopped out of the ambulance and marched with me through the front doors into the school lobby.

"What's with the road barriers being put out this early?" I asked them. "I had to move them to drive in. There aren't any detour signs to mark an alternate route."

"They left one road open but needed to keep the others closed for plowing," responded one of the EMTs.

When we walked in, I could see people bustling around, preparing the reception desk at the entrance, putting army cots in classrooms for staff to sleep on, plugging in the TV in the hallway, and setting up the ever-present coffee pot behind the reception desk. We were greeted with two signs. One gave notice about dealing with the flu, and the other addressed drugs and weapons.

I was always amazed at how a school or a church could be transformed into a disaster shelter in a matter of hours. Many of the staff and volunteers were deployed from other towns and even other states. Most had never worked together before, but Red Cross staff and volunteers were required to take disaster training classes so they worked in precision and harmony in a crisis, knowing exactly what they needed to do and how to do it. If they

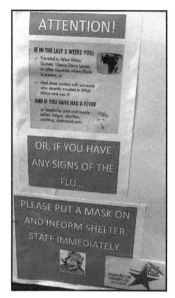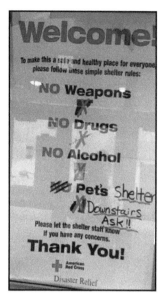

Signs at the shelter entrance.

had a specific assignment, like driving the Emergency Rescue Vehicle (ERV) or functioning as social workers or food handlers, they were required to take additional training. They worked together with a common mission and dedication.

The Cape Cod Disaster Animal Response Team (CCDART) dragged dollies carrying large crates to the elevators to the lower level where they would care for the animals of people who came in. This service was established in 2008 and is partnered with American Red Cross. In the past, people had to leave their animals at home if they wanted to come to the shelters. Many people put themselves in hardship and sometimes in jeopardy because they wouldn't come to the shelters without their animals and some had no choice but to leave their pets alone in homes with no heat. In response to this need, the Federal Pets Act of 2006 required states to plan for the evacua-

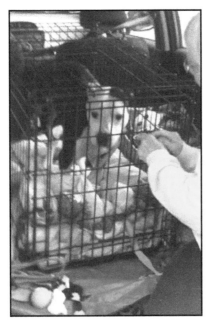

Cape Cod DART Rescue Team caring for animals.

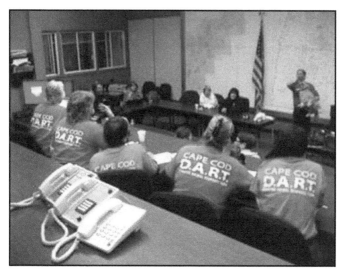

CCDART training session

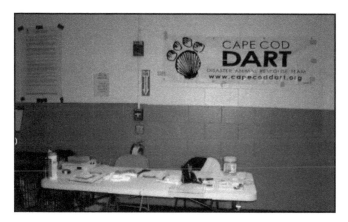

Setting up to receive animals in the shelter
Cape Cod Disaster Animal Response Team,
West Barnstable, MA.

tion of pets during disasters in order to qualify for FEMA reimbursement.

The atmosphere was charged with anxiety and nervous energy as people went about setting up their stations. Given the intensity of activity, I was amazed at how quiet it was. The staff spoke in hushed tones. All of these volunteers had left their families and loved ones to be here to care for those who could no longer stay in their homes, whether because of a power failure, no heat, no way to prepare food, flooding, or needy family members could not be cared for when the roads closed.

I took on this new challenge after working as a nurse for forty years in various Cape Cod hospitals. I decided it was time for a new adventure, and this is what I chose to do when Nemo hit the Cape. I had been volunteering as a nurse for the Red Cross for five years.

The public has very little awareness of what nurses really do. I can't blame them because the "fluff my pillow, bend my straw" portrayal of nurses in the media is often inaccurate and based on outdated concepts of the nurse's role, perpetuating the image of nurses as being the physicians' handmaidens.

Nurses are depicted in TV shows like *Gray's Anatomy*, *E.R.*, *House*, and *Scrubs* as wasting their time having affairs with doctors or hanging around with the EMTs and police drinking coffee. (I have never figured out where that room is that they supposedly sneak into to grab a kiss or a grope or more.)

Then TV came up with *Nurse Jackie*, who was finally depicted as an excellent and competent nurse but, of course, they couldn't leave it at that. They had to make her drug-dependent and cynical. Jackie is hardly a typical nurse.

The media still has difficulty to portray what a modern nurse's life and work really are. After many years of short staffing, too many patients, administrators who only care about the bottom line, shifts that allow no time for nurses to sit down and hardly enough time for them to grab a bite or go to the bathroom — I suppose many nurses might become cynical.

My Red Cross training required me to take classes on the history and background of the Red Cross and how to respond as a nurse in various disasters and sheltering situations.

During that time, I discovered that Clara Barton (her real first name was Clarissa; if I had been called Clarissa, I think I would have changed it to Clara too) was the founder of the American Red Cross. She is often referred to as a nurse, but she wasn't. She was an educator. Nor did she open the first Red Cross headquarters. The Red Cross had been founded in Switzerland in 1866 by Jacob Dubbs, but Miss Barton is credited with bringing it to America.

I was impressed that she was as determined and courageous as Florence Nightingale, and like Nightingale, all of her clinical skills were self-taught. It's not her fault that she wasn't trained as a registered nurse. She was born in 1821, only one year after Nightingale. Education for nurses had not yet been developed. But during her career she did rub shoulders with the likes of Susan B. Anthony and Frederick Douglass, both of whom gave her the inspiration to become a civil rights activist.

I once gazed on a statue erected in her honor when I visited the Red Cross Headquarters in Washington, DC. It stands in the beautiful gardens behind the building.

The truth is that none of the Red Cross classes or training sessions prepared me for what really happens in a shelter. Sheltering is like working in a camp in the middle of a wilderness. There are no doctors to call, no pharmacists to bring in needed medications, no aides to help with the care of the patients, and no one to ask for a second opinion except the nurse I am working with, if there even is one.

There was usually, but not always, a psychiatrist to deal with those who were suffering from the stress of having to leave their homes and an ambulance stays parked outside the door should someone need to be brought to the hospital. But I am on my own with medical decisions and must make do with whatever supplies the Red Cross provided me in a trunk-sized plastic tub.

Often, a Medical Reserve Corps (MRC) nurse is assigned with me. The MRC is a national network of volunteers, organized to help with the health and safety of their communities. Their work is similar to that of the Red Cross. There always seemed to be some confusion as to who is in charge of the shelter medical stations — the Red Cross or the MRC — but we have always worked together and made decisions mutually.

I approached the reception desk and addressed the buttocks of a man bent under the reception table, untangling the wires of the phones he was setting up.

"Where will the health services be set up?"

He peered up over the desk and looked at my Red Cross vest. His eyes moved down the red crosses on my white lanyard to my name tag. Then he stood up and gave me a robust handshake.

"Welcome aboard, Terri. We've been waiting for you. I'm Scott. I work with the EMS (Emergency Medical Services). Follow me."

Scott was a muscular man with glossy black, wavy hair cut close to the sides and a tiny "soul patch" of hair just below his lower lip. His complexion shone from a recent close shave. There was a vein on the left side of his forehead that pulsed. He was a buff, broad-shouldered man who had an air of confidence as he led me down the hallway to a dark, windowless room near one of the classrooms. The desks and chairs it had originally stored were now stacked up on top of each other against the far wall. With only one dim overhead light hanging from the middle of the ceiling, the room had the ambiance of an interrogation room.

"This isn't the nurse's room where I am supposed to be set up, Scott. I've always worked out of the nurse's room where there is an exam table, bathroom, sink, and privacy curtain. There's none of that here."

"Sorry. The shelter manager put you in this room because there are no windows. She was worried that hurricane winds might blow out some of the windows. There's a public bathroom down the hall from here."

I put my bag on the desk and glanced around the room. I pointed to the wall of chairs and tables. "I'll need those chairs to be unloaded and some cots and blankets brought in. Is there a place for me to sleep?"

"Sleep? I don't think you'll be sleeping much with this storm. We'll be bringing everything over, including your cots, as soon as more help arrives. The Red Cross supply tub is over there." He said pointed to a large, blue plastic tub. The lid was snapped shut and closed with adhesive tape. (What would nurses ever do without adhesive tape?)

"We're expecting to be going full boogie tilt when the storm starts knocking out people's electricity."

"And when do you think that will be?"

He looked at his watch. "About supper time."

"What about the power here?"

"Don't worry about it. If it goes out, the back-up generator will kick in. If that happens, you can use any of the red receptacles. Those are connected to the generator."

I put my coat on the back of the chair next to the desk.

"Who is the shelter manager?"

"Pat McNutter. I don't know her because I deployed from New Bedford to here but my guess is that you'll find her in the communications room, where they are setting up the short-wave radios and the telephone system."

I could hear the animated voice of the newscaster coming from the TV in the hallway.

We are anticipating a historic Top 5 snowstorm. White-out conditions will make driving treacherous, so stay off the roads. Governor Deval Patrick has activated 500 members of the National Guard as the blizzard bears down. Marcy Reed, president of National Grid, said power failures could last several days because repairs would require unearthing power lines buried under mounds of snow. The National Weather Service is expecting flooding up and down the Massachusetts coast but especially on the south shores, including Cape Cod.

Then I recognized the Governor's voice.

All MBTA services have been suspended, and roads will be blocked to all but emergency personnel. We have thousands of snowplows and sanders ready for a snow-clearing marathon on interstates and on back roads from Cape Cod to the Berkshires. This is a storm of major proportions. I can't stress this enough.

Please, please stay indoors and off the roads.

I ripped the tape off the Red Cross supply tub and began going through it but stopped when I saw Scott standing in the doorway wheeling an oxygen concentrator with one hand while supporting with the other a man with labored breathing.

"Here's your first patient," he said.

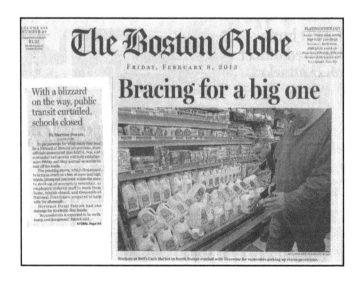

Chapter 2
LET THE FUN BEGIN

2:20pm

I looked for key words on the admission assessment paper Scott handed me and found them.

Name: Manny Mendoza, age 74

Problem: COPD. (Chronic Obstructive Pulmonary Disease) Dependent on his oxygen concentrator. Worried his electricity would be cut off and his oxygen concentrator will stop working.

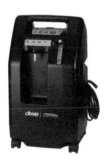

Example of a typical oxygen concentrator (DeVilbiss) Photo from internet (There was no copyright statement.)

I pulled my chair out for him to sit while I plopped myself on the edge of my desk. "Mr. Mendoza, how is your breathing right now?"

He adjusted his oxygen cannula to fit more comfortably in his nose. "I can breathe pretty well as long as I am on my oxygen."

I listened to his lungs and heard the telltale wheeze of a person struggling with COPD or emphysema. His

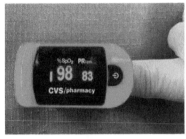

Pulse oximeter or POX.
(Photo courtesy of the author)

blood pressure was slightly elevated at 148/89. I reached into my bag and pulled out my pulse oximeter. It is referred to as a POX meter and measures the patient's oxygen saturation level and pulse. I had asked the Red Cross to include one in their supply bin, but they didn't think it was necessary, so I bought my own for situations just like this.

I placed it on his finger and read the little LED screen, not aware that I was holding my breath until I saw the number 95% pop up.

Then I exhaled. I knew that COPDers did well until they went below 90%. His pulse was slightly elevated at 88, but he was stable.

He eased back into the chair and gave me a "what's next?" look.

"Do you mind waiting a minute? I just arrived and need to get my paperwork out of the supply tub."

He spoke between rasps. "You...you go ahead. I'll just...sit here and catch my breath. That was a long walk from the door to here."

I shuffled though the blue tub of supplies, making a mental note of what was in it. Baby and adult diapers. Packs of sterile gauze. Dressings. Tape. A box with the word "medications" written on a strip of adhesive tape placed across the top. Two stethoscopes. Thermometers, oral and rectal (don't get them mixed up). Alcohol wipes. A bottle of sterile saline and a bottle of alcohol. Cold and hot packs.

I reached for the white notebook filled with the forms I would need to process admission for patients with various problems. As I scanned through the tabs to find the correct admission forms, I noticed one and shuddered: "Deceased" was written across the tab.

"Deceased," I pondered the word. "People actually die in these temporary shelters?" I raised a silent prayer. "Oh, please, God, don't let anyone die on my watch."

I was filling out Mr. Mendoza's admission paper when Scott reappeared, wheeling an IV pole with one hand and steadying an emaciated-looking woman with the other. A feeding bag hanging from the hook on the pole swung back and forth.

"Got another patient," he announced.

As he disappeared out the door, I called out, "Scott, I need someone to unstack these chairs – and bring in some cots!"

"Can't right now," he called back. "Got people lined up at my desk. I'll get an AmeriCorps kid to help you."

I brought over another chair for the woman and sat on the desk again while interviewing her. She was 57 and had undergone surgery for esophageal cancer. Most of her nutrition and hydration came from a milky solution via the feeding tube inserted into her stomach. She was about five feet tall and looked all of about eighty pounds. Her skin hung like drapes from her arms. Her cheeks were sunken. Her voice was weak, almost a whisper. "I live alone, but my daughter comes by every day to flush my tube. I hate making her do that."

"Mrs..." I looked down at her admission paper. "Mrs. LeBlanc..."

"You can call me Nan, for Nancy."

"Okay, Nan. I can help show you how to flush your feeding tube later and then you won't have to wait for your daughter to do it."

"Oh, no. It's very complicated, you know."

"Actually, Nan, it isn't. I promise you that before you leave here you will be flushing out your own feeding tube."

"You are such a dear. I'm a bit chilly. Do you have a blanket?"

I stuck my head out the door to find Scott and saw the growing line in front of his desk.

Another volunteer walked by me. "Can you please get me a blanket for this woman and a few army cots?"

"Yes, ma'am." The boy sported a tumbleweed of red hair that stood upright, defying gravity. He looked to be about 16 years old. Definitely one of the AmeriCorps kids, I thought.

I put my coat around the thin woman and went back to finishing the admission forms for both patients.

The red-headed AmeriCorps kid came in pushing a flatbed cart stacked with folded cots, blankets, and little bags of personal items: soap, toothbrush, and face cloth. "Where do you want me to put these, ma'am?"

"Set up about ten army cots around the room. Put a chair by each of them, a couple of blankets on top, and a bag of personal items on top of the blankets."

"Yes, ma'am."

"My name is Terri. What's yours?" I asked while holding out my hand to him. He met my hand with his.

"Justin, ma'am."

Scott reappeared. "Brought you another patient."

"Wait a minute, Scott. I thought they were sending me another nurse. This makes it three patients in fifteen minutes and we have three more days to go. Can you send the shelter manager in here for me to talk to her?"

30

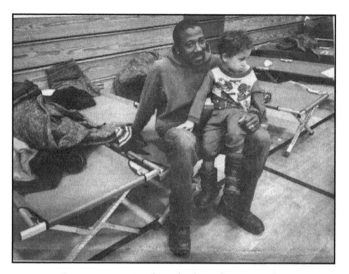

Cots set up in the shelter for people.
Cape Cod Times, February 11, 2013

The voice of the newscaster on the TV outside the room sounded more urgent.

> *We are expecting about 50 to 60,000 of NStar's customers to be without power on the Cape and Islands. People living near the coast have been told to evacuate their homes. Charles Orloff, Executive Director of the Blue Hills Observatory and Science Center, reports that wind gusts will reach up to 80 miles per hour and will cut power*

lines and topple trees. Astronomically high tides are predicted to produce widespread coastal flooding and erosion.

I was processing my third patient, who was also a COPDer and dependent on his oxygen tank, when Scott reappeared. "Pat McNutter, the shelter manager, can't come here to see you. She's too busy setting up communications. She said you'll have to go see her."

"I can't leave three patients alone to go see her. Can you get me the Red Cross representative for the shelter?"

Fifteen minutes later, a trim, short, dark-haired woman in her late thirties showed up and strode toward me with her hand held out. I immediately recognized her as Donna Redburn, the Red Cross manager for this district.

"So this is what you do in your spare time? Aren't you a glutton for punishment," she joked.

I took her hand and held it. "Last time I saw you, you talked me into being the nurse for a basketball game in Boston for underprivileged kids. I was using cold juice boxes as ice packs for bruises and scrapes. It's the only time I ever told someone that once their swelling went down, they could drink their cold pack. What are you doing on the Cape? Not enough to keep you busy in Boston?"

"Same as you. I wondered who would be running the medical clinic." She gave the room a slow sweep. "Now that I know it's you, I can relax. I see you're jumping right in. So what's up?"

"I was told by Alice Kent-Levinson—you know her, right?" Donna nodded yes. "That she would be sending me another nurse, possibly from the Medical Corps. I've gotten three patients since we opened fifteen minutes ago. Usually two nurses work the clinic, especially in a big storm like this one. I tried to reach the shelter manager, but she's busy in the communications room and wants me to come see her. I can't leave these three patients alone to do that. Can you find out if Alice found another nurse and when they will be arriving?"

"Will do." She handed me a card. "And if you need anything, here's my number. I'm setting up the kitchen for supper right now.

Also, a lot of the people will be hanging out there watching the TV. If you can't reach me, get one of the AmeriCorps kids to find me."

I explained where the bathroom was and directed the patients to pick out one of the army cot set-ups for themselves. The two COPDers picked set-ups next to each other but stood staring at the flat beds and didn't sit down.

"I have to stay upright to breathe easy. Do you have any pillows?" Manny asked.

I stepped out into the corridor and yelled over to Scott for pillows.

"No pillows," he called back. "But we'll get you some extra blankets to roll up instead."

The two men agreed that this would be helpful for them.

Within the hour, I had five patients. Donna had not returned with news about another nurse. I picked up the wall phone to try to reach her. The line was dead.

Chapter 3

JAN HOLLOWAY

3:20pm

I was busy finishing the admission paper-work when I heard a pleasant voice coming from the doorway. "Is this where the shelter clinic is? I was waiting in the nurse's room."

I looked up to see a woman sticking her head out from around the edge of the door. She looked to be in her fifties and had short salt-and-pepper hair and a kind smile.

"Yes, such as it is. They wouldn't let me set up in the nurse's room."

She walked over to the desk and let her shoulder bag hit the floor with a thump and in a welcoming manner, reached out with her hand. "I'm Jan Holloway from the Medical Corps. They told me you needed another nurse."

"Frickin' fantastic! I'm Terri Arthur. Am I glad to see you!" I gave her a hug. "Have you ever worked in the shelters before?"

"Every now and then. And you?"

"This is my fourth time."

We reviewed the admissions of the five patients I had checked in. I showed her the supplies we had to work with in the Red Cross tub.

"The Medical Corps will also be bringing in supplies, so we should be well stocked," said Jan.

Then we began the conversation almost all nurses have when they first meet. We usually start with where we went to school. Jan had gotten her degree from Catherine Labouré, a very prestigious nursing school in Boston. She worked at Massachusetts General Hospital and the Visiting Nurses Association (VNA), then took a teaching position at Curry College in Plymouth.

My career took a more circuitous route in that I started my career with a degree in secondary education, with a teaching field of biology, from Bob Jones University in Green-ville, S.C. (Did I like it there? No, I hated it but I got some scholarship loans and needed the money.) After teaching for a year, I decided nursing was a better choice for me and graduated from with a diploma from the Greenville General Hospital, a thousand-bed city hospital. Once I got established professionally on the Cape, I went on to get a masters in Health Business Management from Lesley University in Cambridge, Massachusetts. "So I'm a bit of a hybrid," I told her.

"How was it living in the South?" asked Jan.

"Being a Yankee going to school in the South in the sixties was quite an experience. I felt like I was in a foreign country. The language, customs, culture, food were all so very different from what I had been used to. And they weren't very friendly to 'Northerners.' The interesting part was that I learned all of my medical terms with a Southern accent. So the word femoral came out sounding like fee-moral. I got razzed quite a bit when I started my first nursing position, in the cottage hospital on Martha's Vineyard off Cape Cod."

Just then the feeding machine began to beep. I looked up to see that the bag was empty.

"Hey, Jan. Could you go over and change the bag and reset the numbers on the machine, while I check with Scott to see when those extra cots and blankets will be brought in?"

"Sorry. I can't do that. I don't know anything about those tube feeding machines."

"You don't? What is your specialty?"

"Maternity."

"Maternity?" I asked, hoping I hadn't heard correctly. "So...you haven't done any medical/surgical nursing?"

"I haven't done medical/surgical nursing since I was a student. I just birth the babies. I have done some pediatrics and a lot of community health."

I was speechless. My enthusiasm for having another nurse to help me sank. "Okay now. I'll change the bag, and maybe you can go check on our supplies."

A few minutes later, she came back. "The cots and blankets are being loaded and will be here shortly, Scott said."

She sat pulled a chair out from the stack, brought it to the desk and sat down. "Have you ever worked in maternity?"

"Only when I was floated there. The last time that happened, they assigned me to be the medication nurse on one side of a nursing unit with fifteen patients. There was another nurse and an LPN providing the direct care. I thought that this would be an easy assignment, until I received the eighth request for pain medications and the day shift report was only half done."

"Yup! That's a frequent request. Especially from those who were given C-sections or had an episiotomy."

I continued. "It was the evening shift when the two nurses working on my side said they were leaving for supper. If I had any questions, they said I could ask the nurse on the other side. I was running around answering lights when a patient put on her call light. I went into her room and she asked me, 'When should my baby boy be circumcised?' I had absolutely no idea. 'Good question. I'll get back to you.'

I found the nurse on the other side and asked her. She looked puzzled. 'How would I know? I'm a float here from the outpatient department, where we do colonoscopies and endoscopies, not circumcisions. The other two maternity nurses went to supper together. They told me that if I had any questions to ask the nurse on the other side.'

'I'm the nurse on the other side. I'm from a cardiac telemetry unit. Let's hope all goes well in the next 45 minutes.'

"I waved back to her as I turned back. 'If you need any help, just ask 'the nurse on the other side.'"

"I went back to the mother of the baby boy and said, 'Soon. You should have the circumcision done real soon.'"

Jan laughed at the irony of the situation. "That's how I would feel if they put me on your cardiac unit."

"So tell me, Jan. I never did find out when a male baby does get circumcised."

"Usually 24 to 72 hours after birth. If the baby is Jewish, then it is usually done on the eighth day by a rabbi or a *mohelet,* a religious circumciser. That could even be a Jewish nurse practitioner. In fact, I believe that Alice, your Red Cross head nurse, is one."

"I'm glad that mother didn't wait for me to get back to her. It only took me fifteen years to finally get the answer."

We laughed at my confession; then Jan looked over the admission papers. "So what's next?"

"How about if you get the vital signs and I'll do the admission assessments. You can help monitor the patients after they have been admitted. Anyone under four feet tall will be your patient. If a woman comes in yelling, 'Help! Help! I'm coming!' That's yours too," I joked, then added, "I don't birth the babies and pediatrics is my weakest area, so in a way, it's good that you can cover my weak spots. Is that okay with you?"

"Sure. I'm glad you are here too. Sorry I don't know what to do with that feeding pump," she said, jutting her chin towards the empty bag, then looked over to Manny. "And we never had oxygen concentrators in maternity, but I do remember dealing with them when I was a VNA nurse."

Scott came through the door pushing a woman in a wheelchair. He handed Jan the admission paperwork.

"Hey, Scott. There are no phones in this storage room. How do I call you, the shelter manager, or Donna, the Red Cross person downstairs, when I need something? Can you arrange for one to be hooked up?"

"I'll try. In the meantime you'll just have to rely on your cell phones unless it's AT&T. That won't go through."

"My phone is AT&T. So what's plan B?"

"I guess I'm plan B," said Jan holding up her phone. "I use Verizon."

"Or just stick your head out the corridor and yell," said Scott. "Brace yourself. The next few hours will keep us very busy. The snow is piling up, and the roads will be closed except for emergencies. By supper time, no one will be allowed to drive in unless they call the police to bring them in."

As if on cue, I heard the newscaster's voice.

> The blizzard is bearing down. When you add two respectable storms together, you're going to get a knockout punch. In Southeastern Massachusetts and Cape Cod, wet heavy snow and winds gusting over 75 mph have been reported, forcing hundreds of families to flee to the shelters. The shelters are accepting people in….'

He listed all of the towns and the available shelters.

I went over to Jan, who was taking the vital signs of our new patient. She was barely five feet tall and almost as wide. Well, all right, maybe I exaggerate a bit, but wide enough that she could barely walk, which is why she had been brought in with a wheelchair. Both her legs were edematous and weeping a yellow fluid through gauze bandages wrapped around her lower legs. Her ankles were bright red, a typical symptom of cellulitis or infection. She was 90 years old. We noticed the crotch of her pants was wet. Jan and I looked at each other. We didn't have to say anything. We knew her care would be a challenge in these barest of accommodations.

After admitting her, Jan brought her to the bathroom, cleaned her up, and placed an Attends on her. Then Jan brought the woman over to her army cot.

"I can't sleep on that! I need a bed. I have to have my head up."

"Mrs. Cormier, we don't have beds. This is a high school shelter. I can pile up some blankets for you to lean on."

She became more agitated. "I can't get in and out of that thing. I need a bed. A real bed!"

I asked Jan to find the shelter manager. Fifteen minutes later, she returned with a tall woman with dusty blond hair cut in a pageboy style. She pushed a pair of dark-rimmed glasses up on her nose. She strode into the room with a look of annoyance and confidence that verged on conceit. Tossing her head, she flipped her hair out of her eyes. "I'm Pat McNutter, the shelter manager, and you are...?

"Terri Arthur, the nurse in charge of the medical..."

"Yeah, okay. What is it? Make it quick. I have a phone call to make."

I explained the problem with the recent admission. "She would be safer if she were transferred to the hospital. We don't have a bed for her, and she won't sleep on the cot." I pointed to the woman's swollen, weeping legs. "And she needs treatment for her cellulitis."

"She's not going anywhere. I'll get them to bring you the exam table from the nurse's room."

"The exam table won't do. It's too high and...." She turned on her heels and strode out. She never waited to hear my concern.

"And a hearty hello and welcome to you too," I muttered under my breath.

Two AmeriCorps kids wheeled in the exam table. It was no wider than our patient and was as high as her chest. I had no idea how she would get onto it or off of it. I asked the boys if they knew where there was a stool for her to step up. They said they would try to find one and left.

"I have to go to the bathroom again," shouted Mrs. Cormier. Jan agreed to take her in the wheelchair. As she headed towards the door, I handed her an adult diaper. "You might need another one of these." Jan rolled her eyes to the ceiling, took it from my hand, and gave the wheelchair a shove down the hall. She turned back at me and whispered, "Now I remember why I went into maternity nursing."

Chapter 4
SHE'S MISSING

5:30pm

By 5:30, my patients were asking when supper would be served. I looked down to the reservation desk but couldn't find Scott. An EMT walked by with a St. Bernard mix on a leash. I asked him if he had heard anything about supper.

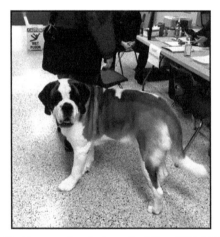

St. Bernard mix headed for CCDART.
(Photo taken by Terri Arthur)

"Nope. I'm heading down to the DART people with Prince here. I'll ask around and get back to you, but you might want to check with the Red Cross lead, Donna Redmond. She's in the cafeteria downstairs."

I headed down a flight of stairs and then walked a long corridor to the cafeteria down the far end of the building. Donna was setting up a table with packaged cookies, chips, and water. Like seagulls facing the wind to keep their bearing, people sat at the tables all facing the TV. I looked at the screen and saw a dark figure on skis emerging from a blurred blizzard of white. An unseen voice from the background said,

All flights in the entire Northeast have been cancelled.

According to the National Weather Service in Taunton, winds are reaching as high as 85 miles per hour in Hyannis and 77 on Nantucket. There are outages all over the Cape, but Mashpee has the highest number. An NSTAR spokesperson reports there is a sheared utility pole down at the Airport Rotary. The number of people who

47

have sought refuge at one of the Cape's four regional shelters has reached 200. Snow totals have reached twelve inches and are predicted to be twice as high by the middle of the night.

I reached into one of the cardboard boxes and helped Donna lay out the cookies and chips. We both worked in silence until I started the conversation. "People are asking about supper."

"We're still waiting for the Emergency Services to bring us our meals," she said as she handed me an armful of snacks. "Take some of these for now, and I'll let you know when the meals arrive."

"My AT&T won't work in this building, so you'll have to call the other nurse, Jan." I handed her Jan's number.

A half-hour later, an AmeriCorps kid arrived with a paper bag in his hand and dumped a dozen bagels on the desk.

"What's this?" I asked.

"It's supper."

"Only plain bagels?"

"Sorry. It's all they could get. The food trucks couldn't make it through. Too many downed lines and trees across the roads."

"No jelly, cream cheese, peanut butter or anything to drink?"

"Nope. This is all they gave me."

In all three of my previous experiences, we were always served a hot meal. It might be lasagna or even pizza with a salad but never just bagels thrown on the desk with nothing but water to drink.

I had a nostalgic flash of what I would be eating if I were home at this time. Elaine had stocked up for a few day's worth of suppers before the storm hit. Tonight she was cooking up a rib-eye steak, a baked potato, and butter-nut squash. I'd be biting into a crusty dinner roll filled with melted butter. We would be sharing a glass of wine together and saving enough room for a piece of Boston cream pie. The fireplace logs would be crackling in the background. She would be complaining that it makes the room too hot and would strip down to a tee shirt. I'd be countering that's it's too cold while I snuggled up in a long, fuzzy bathrobe.

I looked down at the pile of plain bagels. Everyone gathered around the desk and stared at them. They all looked as I did when I was a child and my mother served liver and onions for supper. "It's good for you," she would say as I picked at the overcooked, leathery liver and slithery onions on my plate.

"I know," I'd answer back. "The poor children in China are going hungry. Can I mail this to them?"

"Don't be a smart ass," she always replied.

I brought back the cookies and chips I was able to pick up in the cafeteria. The ten-year-old boy pushed his wheelchair-bound mother up to the table. She looked over the bagels.

"I'm on a gluten-free diet. Is there something else to eat?"

Jan and I gave each other with one of those "Now what?" looks. I offered her my bananas and Jan had some peanut butter cups. We gave them to the woman. I also gave the boy a few packages of chocolate chip cookies.

"I'm a diabetic," said one of the COPDers. "I can't eat a bagel and cookies for supper. It will throw my sugar off."

"We need to call Donna about this."

The word back from Donna wasn't good. She said bagels were all they had been given. She said she would keep trying to bring something more in and would let me know if she succeeded.

Just then I noticed one of the patients was eating out of a tin can. She had a bulging bag of food items that spilled out on her cot. I noticed Spam, miniature hot dogs, tuna fish, crackers, Cheetos. The rest was hidden in the bag.

"Pica," said Jan. "I admitted her. She has an eating disorder. She asked me if she could bring in her cans of food and I told her it would be ok."

"What's her name?"

"Cathy."

"Let's see if we can cut a deal with her."

"Hi, Cathy," I started. "Do you like chocolate chip cookies?"

"Oh yes! Can I have some?"

"I need to give your can of hot dogs to another person. Can we trade?" I held out the cookies to her so she could smell the chocolate. She handed me the tin, never taking her eyes off the cookies.

51

"Okay, but just this once."

"You're great for helping us out. Thank you, Cathy!"

Two more patients checked in. One had cancer and was being treated with chemotherapy, and the other was on crutches and had a bandaged lower leg from an Achilles tendon repair. After I admitted them, I looked up into the room and realized someone was missing.

"Where's Cathy, the woman with pica?" I asked Jan.

"She said she was going to the bathroom but hasn't returned. That was ten minutes ago." Jan rushed out of the door. "I'll check the bathroom." She returned to say the woman wasn't there or anywhere near our station. "She can't be too far away. I'll go find her."

I wrapped blankets around the thin frame of the woman with cancer and set up another chair for the man on crutches to rest his leg on.

Twenty minutes later, Jan returned. "I've been through all of the classrooms that have people in them. I checked the gym and all of the bathrooms. I asked around, but no one has seen her. You don't think she tried to go outside, do you?"

I felt a shadow of fear creeping up the back of my neck. I remembered the tab in the notebook - "Deceased." I tried not to think about it. "Oh, God, no. Please don't let us find her outside in this storm," I said to Jan.

"She left her bag of food," said Jan, pointing to Cathy's army cot. "She wouldn't leave the facility without that."

I went out to the reception desk where most of the support staff seemed to hang out, and explained the situation to everyone there.

"We'll each take a section of the building and start searching for her," said Scott. He put his hand on my shoulder. "Stop worrying, Terri. We'll find her."

"But this is a huge building. Do you think she wandered off or got confused and then lost?"

"We'll keep looking until we find her. You just worry about the people you already have in there."

Chapter 5
MAKE IT WORK

7:30pm

The patients who could walk took their chairs out into the hallway to join the others who sat and watched the progress of the storm on the TV.

> *50,000 homes are without power on the Cape. Phone companies are preparing for cell tower power outages. Verizon Wireless reports they have at least eight hours of backup power to all of its cell towers. Their technicians are busy making sure their generators will kick in once the batteries are depleted. AT&T and Sprint are making similar preparations. Marissa Shorenstein, the president of AT&T reports, "With a storm of this magnitude, we have to be ready to activate back-up power as soon as possible."*

I checked my watch: 7:30pm. I knew it would be a very long night. Just then, Donna came up the stairs holding Cathy's arm. "Is this the woman you were looking for? I found her in the cafeteria kitchen. She was going through the refrigerators and cabinets. She said she was hungry and looking for food."

Donna took the bag the pica woman was carrying and dumped it on the table. Out tumbled a half-dozen yogurt containers, a few dry cereal boxes and pint-sized milk cartons, and sample-sized containers of peanut butter.

"Hey! Leave those alone. Those are mine! I found them!" protested the woman as she scooped everything back into the bag and ran over to her cot.

I went down to the kitchen to ask Donna if she could keep her new food stash. Donna held her hands up in a gesture of submission. "She has already handled this food so I can't put them back. But please keep her out of the kitchen. That food isn't ours. It belongs to the school. We have to account for everything that is missing."

After Donna left, I turned to Jan. "Hey, look at the bright side. We now know what we can do if they don't bring us enough food. We'll just set her loose to raid the kitchen."

But Cathy wasn't going to part with her new stash of food. "They are all mine. I found them," she protested when I asked if she would be willing to give up a few yogurts.

"How about if we trade some peanut butter cups for three of the yogurts? And I have three bags of potato chips to trade for three of the milks and boxes of cereal. That will still leave you with plenty of food left over."

"I told you I wasn't going to do this."

"I know, but these people are very hungry, and they would really like to have something to eat. Please, can you help us out?"

She hesitated but reached into her bag and handed a few of her prized food possessions to me and I handed her the promised exchange. We then offered them to the patients, who instantly snatched them from my hands.

With the storm raging and the snow piling up in the roads, I knew that at this point people would find it difficult to travel to the shelter. The eight patients we had would be a stable number until the snowplows could clear the roads. There were at least 50 non-patients relaxing in various classrooms. DART had three dogs, one cat, and a gerbil in their downstairs holding area. I secretly envied them. I thought about how much fun it would be to ride out the storm petting and caring for a few friendly dogs and cats.

We asked the mother of the ten-year-old boy if we could bring him over to the gym, where some of the staff were playing basketball. She agreed.

"I can't leave my mom," said the boy. "I have to take care of her. She needs me to be with her." I promised him I would take good care of his mom and not to worry.

"He's such a good boy," said the mother. "You go ahead and play with the other boys. I'll be fine here with the nurses."

We asked one of the AmeriCorps kids to stay with him until he was ready to come back.

She watched him disappear out of the room and turned to me. "When I was diagnosed with MS a few years ago, my husband abandoned me and left me to care for myself and my son. I can walk a little, but it has gotten worse over this past year. I know I will soon be stuck in this wheelchair most of the time. Jack pushes me around. I don't know how I would manage without him."

"You are a saint," I said. "We do have a social worker at the Red Cross. If you need some help, give us a call." She gave my hand a squeeze and then joined the others watching TV in the hallway.

Jan took the 90-year-old woman to the toilet and changed her diaper. The fluid oozing from both of the woman's lower legs had soaked through her dressings. With the help of the step stool the Americorps kid found for us, we helped her get up on the exam table that would be her bed for the night.

She sat on the edge while Jan supported her and I changed the dressings. It was then that we both saw that there was an obvious problem. She was at risk of rolling off the edge of the narrow exam table in her sleep. There were no rails or sides to prevent this from happening.

Jan called the shelter manager on her cell asking her to please come over and help us solve this problem. The truth was that she should have been transferred to the hospital

ER. We were not prepared to safely care for this woman. Then there was the issue of her cellulitis in both legs oozing infectious drainage over the exam bed and wheelchair.

Pat strode into the room. With both hands, she flipped her hair behind her ears. "What's up?" We showed her the problems we were having.

"She's not safe here, Pat. She's a fall risk waiting to happen, and those legs should be seen and treated by a physician."

Pat was unmoved by our pleas. "She's here now, and it's your job to care for her."

"But it's also our job to triage patients we feel would be unsafe in these basic conditions. She's at risk of breaking her hip or hitting her head. Either would be devastating for this woman."

Pat folded her arms over her chest. "I'm not moving her out until she is ready to go home or someone comes to get her. The rest is up to you. Make it work. You're the nurse." With that, she marched out.

"We can't sit by her bed all night," said Jan. I knew she was right. I looked around the room, desperately trying to find something, anything, that would help us solve this problem. Then I noticed a pile of chairs in the corner stacked on top of each other. "What if we put the exam table against the wall and stacked these chairs higher than the exam table facing outward. The backs would act as bedrails. We could tie them to the table with a rope. If she tried to get up or roll over, she would hit the backs of the chairs and wake up."

It seemed to be the only solution we could come up with. We hoped it would work. Once it was set up, and the patient was settled in, we nervously kept glancing over to her makeshift crib to be sure she was where she was supposed to be.

I now had a few minutes to work with the frail woman with the feeding tube. I wrapped an extra blanket around her and sat next to her. "How about if we flush your feeding tube together?"

"I live alone, but my daughter comes by every day after work to help me with this." She pointed to the place where her feeding tube was inserted into her stomach.

"Sometimes, I can shut it off if I have to go somewhere, like shopping or the doctor's, but I mostly keep it on."

I asked her if I could call her by her first name, Betty. She agreed. "Would you like to learn how to flush this to keep it clear?"

She shook her head. "I don't think I can. I watch my daughter do it and it seems like it's too much for me to remember."

"Let's give it a try. You can't hurt anything."

I reached for the 50cc syringe with the plastic tip that narrowed at the end and showed her how to draw up sterile water into it from a clean cup. I had her pinch the tubing when I removed the feeding line and open up the tubing when I had the syringe in place.

"OK, now. You push the water into the stomach tube." Her hands shook as she worked the plunger on the syringe, but she managed to flush the tube.

"You did it perfectly!" I encouraged her. "Now insert the feeding tube back into the stomach tube." She did as I instructed her. "Well done!"

A smile came over her face. "Now the next time we do this, I'm going to watch and you will do it all by yourself."

"Did I really do it right?"

"Absolutely."

"My daughter will be so happy that I can do this. I can't wait to show her." There was a shiver in her voice. "It's still a bit cool in here. Can you bring me another blanket?"

I was wrapping another blanket around her bony legs and up to her chest when I saw Jan motioning for me to come over to the desk. She was talking to Cathy, the pica woman.

"We have a problem. Cathy here has to lie sitting up near an outlet because she uses a CPAP machine at night."

I checked around the room. One plug was being used by the COPDer who was dependent on his oxygen concentrator machine. The other plug was in use for the feeding machine. We found a third one behind a row of chairs stacked up but needed an extension to make Cathy's CPAP machine reach the outlet.

Then Jan found an outlet in the hallway just outside the door to our room. None of these outlets were red, meaning if the electricity went off, they would not be connected to the back-up generator. We hoped to hell that the electricity would not go off.

We brought Cathy's cot over to the third outlet and stacked a pile of blankets at the head for her to be able to lie with her head and chest upright. Then we brought over all of her bags and piled them at the foot of the cot. I asked Scott to please find me an extension cord so we could bring her back into the room.

Everyone seemed to be settled but Cathy. The extension cord we needed couldn't be found.

I turned to Jan. "We have no choice. Without the extension cord, we will have to move all of the chairs and desks away from the closet for her to reach the outlet."

After moving and stacking them against another wall, we were able to set up Cathy's sleeping quarters with her CPAP machine functioning.

I thought we could finally relax a little when I looked up to see a man standing in the doorway. He had his admission papers in his hand.

"Is this the medical clinic where I check in?"

I motioned for him to come on in. He handed me his papers. It read:

> New onset of cough.
> Slight fever.
> Runny nose and congestion."

Jan took his temp. It was 101.4. I listened to his chest and heard wheezing and congestion.

"How long have you had these symptoms?" I asked.

"About two days, but it's getting worse today."

"Has anyone around you recently had the flu?"

"My grandson visited yesterday but left when we heard about the storm. I know he had a cold."

"Have you had a flu vaccination?"

"I hate those things. They aren't any good anyway. Last year's was only good for seventeen percent of the time. Did you know there's mercury in that stuff and it can cause Alzheimer's?"

Jan and I gave each other a knowing look. The same old arguments against vaccines.

"Shit! He has the flu," I thought to myself. "That's all we need right now."

We knew we had to isolate him from the rest of the population. Jan handed him a mask and a box of Kleenex and took him outside the room while she looked for another place to keep him isolated.

Twenty minutes later, Jan returned. "Well, I have good news and bad news."

"What's the good news? I need good news."

"We found an empty classroom away from everyone else."

"What's the bad news?"

"It's down another hallway far enough away that we will have a problem keeping an eye on him."

"Great. And with the flu, we can't have an AmeriCorps kid stay with him either."

"Does he have a phone?"

"Yes, but it's on AT&T."xxx

"Then we'll just have to make routine rounds to check on him and hope to hell he stays put and doesn't spread it around."

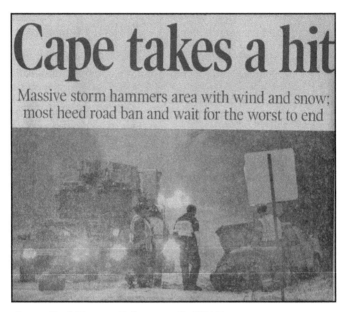

Cape Cod Times, February 9, 2013.

Chapter 6
THE NEWSPAPER REPORTER

8:45pm

Since all our patients seemed to be settled in their places, I asked Jan if she felt comfortable enough to watch them while I checked the weather outside and got some updated news about the storm. I could hear the wind moaning and howling like Marley's ghost around the corner of the building. The windows strained against the blasts of the wind.

A lot can be learned from terrifying storms. Not only are they frightening but also deeply humbling. They represent the power of nature, uncontrolled by humanity, filled with a force that is unstoppable and unforgettable.

I went to the front doors and looked out into a surrealistic scene in the parking lot. Everything was a blinding white. A fearless wind sculpted the tops of the snow piles and then changed direction and re-sculpted them into a different formation. The wind whistled a tune that was beguiling and fearsome at the same time. It reminded me of the Sirens in Greek mythology, creatures who were half bird and half woman and lured sailors to destruction with their beautiful songs.

All areas of recognition were wiped out. I couldn't distinguish where the street ended and the sidewalks began. It could have been a scene taken in the Alaskan or Siberian tundra. Snowdrifts made the parked cars look like hibernating albino behemoths. The only sign of civilization was an abandoned snowplow stuck in the middle of the driveway. Navigating this terrain would have been impossible, and yet I heard the Siren's call of temptation and the desire to risk walking out into this other world to be a part of its strength and beauty.

Scott's voice behind me shook me from my trance. "It broke down. Couldn't handle the snow."

I turned to face him.

"Now we can't plow out the driveway until we can get it towed or they can bring in another plow. We tried to keep the driveway cleared but as soon as we were done, it covered back over again," he said.

I asked him the latest news about the storm.

"They are calling this storm 'monumental' and say the winds will continue at hurricane speed throughout the night. The entire Cape is on lockdown. We're all safe right now but we are concerned about the building's generator. If we lose electricity and have to use it for any extended time, it may not last for the entire storm unless the power kicks back in. They are looking for another generator to back up this one."

"How long do we think this will keep up?"

He ran his fingers through his mop of thick black hair. "It's a nor'easter, so that means it could last as long as three days. The National Grid has sent in additional crews to deal with the blackouts."

He turned to a woman standing quietly behind him and motioned for her to step forward. "We have a newspaper reporter here who has been interviewing some of the staff and people who are sheltering here. She said she was saving the best for last and wanted to talk to Jan and you about the medical clinic."

"That's okay with me, and I'm sure Jan will also talk to her. We just can't have her take pictures of the patients without their permission."

"Jan already knows her. She's featured Jan in other disaster articles."

"Featured her? Why?"

"Because of who she is."

"Who is she?"

"Jan is the Director of the Cape Cod Medical Corps for Barnstable County. She's the head nurse of the organization."

"She's the what?"

"She's the head nurse of the Medical Services," he repeated. "And she was also the former Team Commander at the Department of Homeland Security."

I was stunned.

We walked over to the room where we had set up. When the reporter saw Jan, she dropped her bag on the floor and her camera on the desk and gave her a bear hug. "We have to stop meeting like this," she said to Jan.

"Don't you have enough sense to stay home in this kind of weather?" joked Jan.

"No more than you do, my friend."

"You could at least have told me you were coming and brought us a couple cups of coffee – and doughnuts."

The two of them sat down and spoke like old friends – sharing, teasing, and laughing together. They reminisced about other shelter assignments during storms, fires, and floods. It was obvious that Jan was no stranger to disasters. I felt a wave of guilt wash over me for thinking she wasn't up to the challenge. As it turned out, she was not only experienced in shelter medical care, but also in charge of training and deploying nurses to the various disaster sites.

She turned the reporter's attention to me. "This is my friend, Terri Arthur. She's a nurse sent here by the Red Cross. If you ever need a good nurse, she's the one to call."

The reporter gave me a polite smile, asked me a few routine questions about how the clinic was set up, and then turned back to Jan. She asked Jan about the number of patients we had and what their needs were. She asked the COPDer if she could take his picture for the *Shelton Enterprise* and the patient agreed.

The reporter then picked up her bag and hoisted it up on her shoulder. "I'm bunked down in a classroom that is set up for the shelter staff just down the hall. Stop by. Right now I'm going down to the DART team to see how they are managing with the critters. I hear they have a beautiful St. Bernard mix down there. Now that I know you are here, I know the medical clinic is in good hands."

When she left, I turned to Jan. "I didn't know you were the Director of the MRC. Why didn't you tell me?

"I thought you already knew. What difference does it make? We all have a job to do."

"But you could have sent any one of your nurses over here. Instead, you took the post."

"All of my nurses were already assigned to one of the other four shelters when Alice called for one more nurse, so I agreed to take this assignment. Like the Red Cross, we just don't have enough nurses for disasters like this. In fact, that's why they only opened up four shelters and not the full six. And also, many of our volunteers have gone south for the winter, just like the ones who work with the Red Cross on the Cape."

I suddenly had a mental picture of them sitting by the docks with a piña colada in one hand while the other hand smoothed sunscreen over their legs. How I envied them.

I had always been puzzled about how the emergency service worked on the Cape. Here was my opportunity to finally figure it out. I asked Jan to explain how it worked. "I always thought these shelters were run by the Red Cross."

"It's different on the Cape than anywhere else in the state. We have a Regional Emergency Service Committee (RESC) that is in charge of all emergencies on the Cape. They are funded by the Department of Public Health."

"And where does the DPH get its funding from?" I asked while unfolding the blankets.

"They get it from the federal department of Health and Human Services. The DPH creates a response team of everyone who would be necessary during a disaster. So that would be the police, firefighters, EMTs, health agents, Red Cross, hospitals, Visiting Nurses, Medical Reserve Corps, Salvation Army – about twelve in all. The Cape Cod RESC currently maintains a database of over 300 volunteers from across Cape Cod. We meet once a month."

"And what is the purpose of these meetings?"

"We make sure every town has an emergency manager and is prepared to meet the needs of their town during an emergency. Each town makes its own rules. For instance, just a few years ago, there was a fire chief in Shelton who refused to let the Red Cross be a part of emergency planning in his town."

"Why would he do that?"

"Because ... because ... I don't really know. He used the MRC for nurses instead of the Red Cross. That's all I know."

"Well, that explains why I was never sent to my own town when they opened up the shelters for a disaster."

"It also explains why the Red Cross has so few nurses from your town. I'll bet they were glad to see you walk in the door. Many of the volunteers here have been deployed from other areas of Massachusetts because the Cape is predicted to get the worst impact of this storm."

"So..." I wanted to say this delicately. "The shelter manager here—Pat McNutter. What department is she under, and how did she get the job managing this shelter?"

"Now, that's an interesting question. I honestly don't know. She has never shown up at any of the monthly RESC meetings, and no one has ever mentioned her name. That I know of, she's not a member of any of the departments under the RESC."

"And as far as you know, she has no medical or emergency training or any training for anything related to this shelter?"

"As far as I know, none."

Phone companies prepare cell towers for power outages

By PETER SVENSSON
THE ASSOCIATED PRESS

NEW YORK – Phone companies topped off fuel at cell-tower generators in Northeastern states Friday, preparing for a storm that could bring power outages, and with them, a loss of cell service.

Cell-towers are dependent on electric power from the grid, but many of them have backup batteries, and in some cases generators that can power the antennas independently for longer. Prolonged power outages, such as those after Superstorm Sandy, can bring down cell service in an area.

Verizon Wireless prides itself on having at least eight hours of backup power at all its cell towers, and spokesman Tom Pica said technicians were busy making sure the generators that kick in once batteries are depleted had fuel.

"We also contract with local (fuel) suppliers to ensure regular deliveries if there are extended commercial power issues, as we did during Sandy to positive effect," Pica said.

AT&T Inc. and Sprint Nextel Corp. were making similar preparations, and lining up portable generators to truck out to cell towers with no permanent generators.

"With a storm of this magnitude, we may have some outages. But if service goes down, we'll do all we can to get it back up as fast as possible," said Marissa Shorenstein, president of AT&T New York.

The companies also have "mobile cell towers" – trucks

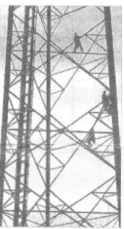

STEVE HEASLIP/CAPE COD TIMES FILE
Preparations for the storm include phone companies making sure backup generators at cell towers have been topped off with gasoline.

that can act as replacement antennas.

Landlines are less susceptible to power outages. The lines carry all the power corded phones need to function, and phone companies have massive battery banks and generators to back them up. Cordless phones won't work without power, though. Phone service from cable companies is also dependent on power, but most companies supply backup batteries to power phones for some hours. Verizon's "FiOS" fiber-optic landline service is also dependent on power and backup batteries.

Cape Cod Times, February 9, 2013.

Chapter 7
THE BACK-UP GENERATOR

J an and I set up a couple of cots for ourselves near the desk and agreed to take turns sleeping and watching the patients. I asked her if I could use her phone to make a few calls while she settled in.

I called my sister first. "Hey, kiddo. Do you still have electricity?"

"It's wild out here," she said. "But everything is going well. The lights keep flickering on and off so I won't be surprised if we soon lose power. If we do, the generator will kick in. We have the gas fireplace on so it's cozy."

"Yeah, our gas fireplace is keeping things cozy here too," I laughed. "The lights have been going off here for a few seconds, but we also have a back-up generator just in case."

"How's the food?" she asked.

"Ha! Food? What food? They dumped a bag of bagels on the table for supper. I'll tell you about it when I get home."

"And when will that be?"

"Not for a while, that's for sure."

"Just get home safe."

"You stay safe too, kiddo."

Next, I called Elaine. She assured me everything was going well enough but that the she feared that the power might cut out. I told her not to worry, because the automatic generator would kick in.

"That means you'll have heat and lights. The refrigerator will stay on and you can still cook on the gas stove. You can also put the gas fireplace on. Boy, that sounds good right now!"

"Do you have to go to these shelters every time there's a storm? I don't like you being out there. Why not let someone else open the medical clinic?"

"Because there is no one else. It's what I signed up to do. I'm okay. Stop worrying. Warm up in front of that fireplace and think of me." I gave her Jan's phone number and told her to call me if there was a problem.

"Promise me you'll get back in the morning."

"I can't promise you that unless Alice , the Chief Nurse of our local Red Cross chapter, finds another nurse to take my place or they close the shelter. From the looks of it, I don't think either will be a possibility. We are almost full. I'll let you know if I hear anything. Now get some sleep."

"I can't sleep until you come home and neither can Jackson. He keeps pacing around looking for you. He is curled up on the couch where you sit and watching the door."

"Then all three of us will be pretty tired because I don't think I'll be sleeping much either. Give our sweet kitty a kiss for me, and save one for yourself. Night. Night."

I asked Jan if she had called her husband. "How does he handle it when you go out on these disasters?"

"Oh, he hates it and tells me he wants me to quit. But he knows this is what I want to do and nags me less now. And you?"

"My sister hates that I do this and my partner, Elaine, tries to talk me out of it too. I think that only nurses understand what nurses do and why we do it."

Nurses, like police and firefighters and anyone who serves the public on a 24-hour basis, often feel the pull between family and what their job requires of them.

"Elaine worked as a medical secretary in the recovery room at the Faulkner Hospital so she knows what it's like to be around nurses. But she's only been living on the Cape for a year and isn't used to the frequent power outages. That's why I had the automatic generator installed."

I settled in on the army cot and had just closed my eyes when I heard a thud. The ceiling light flickered a few yellow rays of light, and then we were shut down in total darkness. I swung my legs over the edge of the cot and held my breath.

"Please God, make that generator kick in," I prayed to myself.

Suddenly a deep rumble came up from the bowels of the building as the back-up generator turned over a few times and then started. A few hallway lights flickered on, but our room and the bathrooms were in darkness. I searched the blue tub for flashlights and found one. Jan found another in her supplies. The oxygen concentrator, the feeding pump, and the CPAP machine fell silent.

I jumped up. "We have to find three red outlets for these patients."

Jan was already on her feet. "There should be someone in charge of the building maintenance out there who knows where the red outlets are. You check out the area and look for the closest red outlets. I'll try to find the maintenance guy."

I went to each patient and told them everything was being handled and not to worry. At the same time, I hoped to hell that Jan would be back soon with some news about where the functioning outlets were. The woman with the feeding pump would be safe for a while, and the CPAP user would just have to sit up and stay awake, but Manny, the COPDer, depended on his oxygen concentrator to supply him with life-sustaining oxygen. Without it, he could deteriorate in a short period of time. I put the oxygen oximeter on his finger. It still read that his oxygen saturation level was 95%, but I knew that wouldn't last. The other COPDer, Joe, would be safe because he had his own oxygen tank.

Fifteen minutes seemed like an hour before Jan returned with the school maintenance man. He looked around the room, scratching his head. "Well, I know there's one in here somewhere or at least near here."

"One?"

"Yeah, one. This was a storage room so they never needed to put more than one here. Some of the people are moving up into the gym. There's more red outlets over there."

"Where's the gym?"

"It's upstairs over in the other building."

"I can't send patients that far away," I protested.

He inspected every wall in the room but couldn't find any of the outlets we needed. Then he looked into the back of the closet where Cathy, the pica woman, had been set up.

"Yup, found it," he said, pointing to a plug in the back of the closet. "And there's another one in the hallway between your room and the bathroom."

I looked into the deep closet filled with electrical switches and wires. "Do you have an extension cord?"

He said he would try to find one and disappeared.

After discussing with Jan who would get which red outlet, we put Manny's army cot and oxygen concentrator partially in the doorway of the closet. His own cord and plug reached to the back of the closet to the red outlet. We also had the red outlet in the hallway. Who would need it the most? Cathy, the pica woman with the CPAP machine or Mrs. LeBlanc with her feeding tube?

"Mrs. LeBlanc said she could go without being fed for a few hours. But I hate to put Cathy out in the hallway where we wouldn't be able to monitor her. She could escape to the kitchen before we realized she's missing."

But we had no choice and moved her cot, bags and CPAP machine out into the hallway.

"It's cold out here," she protested. I gave her another blanket. At least we had plenty of those.

"I'm not sleeping here. There's no privacy, and the light is in my eyes. I can't sleep like this."

I explained that we had no choice. If she wanted to use the CPAP, she would have to stay in the hallway to plug it in.

"It has to be on or I'll stop breathing at night."

"That's right. And that's why you'll have to stay here next to a special plug for power to your machine."

Because of her eating disorder, she had put on a substantial amount of weight. People who are that heavy often have problems breathing while lying down, so they sleep with their heads up and connected to a CPAP machine to help them breathe.

I remembered once taking care of an obese man in the ICU. We couldn't wean him off the ventilator. Within a few minutes of being disconnected from the machine, he would deteriorate and we would have to reconnect him. This went on for days.

Then a long-forgotten little tidbit of information found its way back into my thoughts. *Pickwickian syndrome*. It was named after the obese boy described in Charles Dickens's *The Pickwick Papers*. The boy was unable to lie flat because the weight of his chest and abdomen pressed on his lungs, creating a hypoventilation problem, and he would stop breathing.

With that in mind, we sat our ICU patient bolt upright before we tried to wean him off the ventilator, and it worked. Put him flat and he stopped breathing; sit him straight up and he breathed just fine.

I was pretty sure that Cathy was Pickwickian enough to stop breathing when she lay down to sleep and that was why she used the CPAP machine at night. This was even more of a reason to keep her where we could watch her, but I had no choice. This was the closest place I could put her unless the maintenance man came back with a long extension cord.

"I'm sorry," I said to her. "I know this is difficult and isn't a very good place to try to sleep, but for now it's the only place I have for you. We'll keep checking up on you."

Cathy bunched up her blanket/pillows and leaned back on them. "I'll be waiting for you. This is a scary place to be in the middle of a storm, but I know you and the other nurse will take care of me. Right?"

"Right. If anything changes, we will tell you."

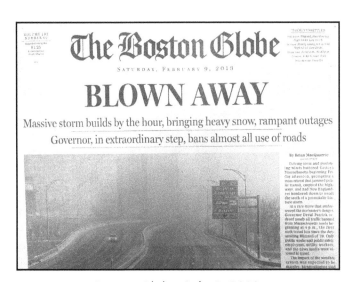

Boston Globe, Feb. 9, 2013

Chapter 8
POWER FAILURE

12:15am

When everyone was tucked in and quiet, I went down to the cafeteria to see the latest news on the one TV that was still functioning. The one in the hallway had ceased to work when we functioned on the back-up generator. The weather forecaster, covered in a fur-lined parka, gave his report while standing in a blur of white. An icy wind could be heard howling like a lonely wolf behind him.

> Driving snow and punishing winds are battering Eastern Massachusetts. This storm is truly one for the record books. Throughout the Northeast, more than 600,000 homes and businesses have lost electricity. Airlines canceled more than 5,300 flights through Saturday, and New York City's three major airports and

Boston's Logan Airport closed. Officials readied snow removal crews with more than 250,000 tons of salt. NStar went on its highest alert. Sadly, in Boston, a 13-year-old boy and a man died separately due to carbon monoxide poisoning while inside cars because the tailpipes were blocked by snow.

Donna came over from the staff room and sat next to me. She handed me a bottle of water. "You'd better get some sleep," she said.

"I can't sleep. This army cot is worse than sleeping on the floor, and I'm worried about the patients I have. They are all a little frightened, especially now that the power has quit. I'm going to have to figure out who gets the two red outlets I have available to me."

"There are at least a half-dozen red outlets in the gymnasium," she said as she read the last weather reports on her cell phone.

"But that's too far from where I am stationed, and I have to be available for anyone else who comes in. Besides I have a few patients who I think should have never been admitted but should have instead been sent directly to the hospital. I can't get McNutter to budge about this. Do you know who she is? No one else seems to know."

"Never saw her before. But if I can help out, let me know. I'm going to try to get some sleep myself."

After watching the news long enough to know what the weather was like out in the cold, cruel world, I returned to our storage room and threw a few blankets across my canvas army cot. Jan was stretched out on hers and tucked under a few blankets.

"I'll take the first few hours watch," I told her. "You try to get some rest."

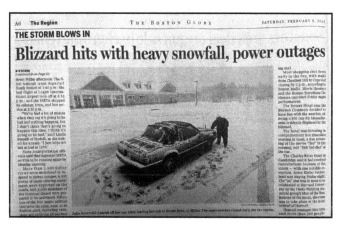

Boston Globe, February 9, 2013

I made a round to check in on everyone. Cathy, the CPAP woman, was still on her cot, and the 90-year-old woman was snoring. Manny maintained his POX at 95% so I checked on the man with the flu. He was turned on his side and asleep. The man with the leg cast was sitting up and reading by flashlight. Then I heard another clunk. We were once again thrust into utter darkness. I waited for the whirr that meant the backup generator had restarted, but heard nothing. I woke up Jan.

"Hey, we're in trouble. The power is off and the generators aren't kicking in. That means the red outlets aren't working. I'm going out to find McNutter to see what is happening and to let her know our situation. Here's the POX. Keep a watchful eye on our COPDers."

I ran to Scott and asked him where Pat McNutter was. "She's in the communications room talking to the maintenance man." I asked him if he knew anything about getting the generators to work. He didn't. I went to the communications room and found McNutter in a heated argument with the maintenance man. I waited until there was a lull in their conversation.

"Pat, I have three patients that need power. One has COPD and needs power to his oxygen concentrator. Another patient is on a feeding tube, and a third can't breathe without her CPAP machine while lying down." We need to transfer these patients to the hospital, especially the one with COPD who is dependent on his oxygen concentrator.

Pat looked at me as if I were a meaningless annoyance. "I've spoken to the maintenance man, and he said the generator will come back on in five minutes, so settle down. I'm not transferring anyone to the hospital."

"But what if it doesn't come on? Then we have lost precious time for a man who won't be able to breathe."

"It. Will. Come. On." She gave me a dismissive look, flipped her hair out of her eyes, turned away, and walked out of the room.

I went back to the room and told Jan about the conversation. "Jan, I'm a nurse. I've handled many bedpans. I can recognize bullshit when I see it."

Jan looked serious. "We can clean bed-pans, but we can't generate oxygen. I checked the other man's oxygen tank and guess what? It's low. He will run out of oxygen in about three hours."

"Damn!" I said a little too loudly. "We'll give McNutter five minutes. Keep checking their POX. If Manny's oxygen drops down to 90%, he's in trouble. We need to call someone about this now. In fact, I think I'll call my nurse manager and let her know about our situation.

I fished around in my pocket for Betty's number. It was 12:00 md. I knew she wouldn't like being called up in the middle of the night, but hell, too bad, I had no choice. Jan handed me her phone, and I dialed Betty's number. It rang four times, five times, six times, and then an answering machine came on. I tried not to sound panicked while leaving the message, but she needed to know we were in a dangerous situation. Then I waited for her to call me back.

Cathy, the pica lady, walked over to me, fishing into her food bag. "I can't sleep with-out my CPAP machine."

I tried to sound calm. "I know, Cathy, but the power is off again. They are working on getting the generator to start back up. If you want to, why don't you come back into the room until it is running again. It's not as cold in here."

"Can I eat my peanut butter crackers?"

"Of course."

Five minutes passed, and the generators still had not kicked in. I placed the oximeter on Manny's finger. It was now 93%. He wasn't in trouble, at least not yet, but I felt like we were playing Russian roulette with his need for oxygen. I went back to look for McNutter and found her sitting at the reception desk.

"The generator isn't on. My patient's oxygen concentration is dropping. We need to transfer him out. And one more thing. The other man doesn't have enough oxygen in his tank to last until the morning. He needs to be sent out as well."

She didn't look up. "We're working on it. It will come on."

"When? One man needs oxygen now, and the other man's tank will be empty in a few hours."

"Soon. Please stop bothering me. You and the others are not the only ones in this shelter." She waved the back of her hand as if shooing an annoying fly. "I said we're working on it."

I went back to Jan. "I'm calling Betty back and will keep calling her every five minutes unless the power comes on." I dialed Betty's number again. It rang until the answering machine came back on. "That's it! She's not answering. I'm calling Alice. What's Manny's last POX?"

"92%."

"If he gets down to 90%, maybe we can implement a buddy system and have him share the other man's oxygen tank. Or maybe we can get another oxygen tank from the EMTs in the ambulance outside."

Suddenly, as I was dialing Alice, I heard a thunk and a whirr. The hallway lights flickered a yellow glow and then brightened. The generator was working! Over the next few minutes, Manny's O2 saturation began to rise to 94% and then back to his normal of 95%.

When Cathy saw the hallway lights come on, she went back to her cot again and strapped on her CPAP mask.

Relieved our emergency was over, Jan and I clinked our water bottles together in a gesture of victory and took a long drink.

Chapter 9
FUNCTIONING WITHOUT OXYGEN

3:00am

At 3:00am, Jan agreed to stay awake while I tried to settle in on the narrow army cot for a few hours of sleep. I had never slept on one before, and after this experience, I hoped I never had to do it again. The canvas was cold and if I bent my knees, they hit the cold metal bars on the edge of the cot. I threw a blanket over the top to protect myself from hitting the metal sides. They were still hard. I soon realized that the only way to sleep on one of these things was to lie on my back with legs straight out. This was going to be a long night.

Just as I was dozing off, Jan woke me up. "The woman on the exam table needs to go to the bathroom and have her Attends changed. I'll need your help." Together, we untied the chairs we had set up as a bed rail, and with each of us holding one of her arms, we slowly eased her down and into a wheelchair. Once we got her into the bathroom and onto the toilet, I saw that her leg dressings were saturated. "We will have to change her dressings. We can do it when we get her back into the room and while she's still in the wheelchair."

Wheeling her back, we saw Scott at the reception desk leaning over a short-wave radio. When he saw us walking over to him, he turned the volume up a bit for us to hear.

Power outages have plagued the Cape. As of 1:15am, about 24,000 NStar customers are without power. Wind gusts are over 80 mph. Woods Hole, Martha's Vineyard, and Nantucket have all cancelled ferry service for tomorrow. Storm surges have created flooding in some areas as this massive storm hammers the area. Emergency services are asking people to shelter in place and wait for the worst to end. More about this as the details come in.

Scott looked up. "They're missing a 90-year-old man who went out looking for his dog and hasn't returned."

"Oh, no. He can't walk with the snow this high. He may have gotten disoriented in the snow and lost his way back."

"Could be. He's been missing for four hours now so it doesn't look good."

We wheeled our 90-year-old woman back into the room, lifted her onto the exam table, and tied the chairs back around her "bed." We still had to do something about the fact that one of our COPDers had a tank with only a few hours of oxygen left in it.

I went back to look for McNutter. She was sitting in the communications room with her feet up on the desk, drinking coffee. When she saw me, she folded her arms and leaned back against her chair. "Pat, the COPDer with the O2 tank will soon be out of oxygen. We have to either evacuate him or get him an oxygen tank from the EMT's ambulance."

I now realized that she seemed to wear a perpetual sneer on her face. "I'm not going to bother them now," she said as she sipped her coffee. "And I'm not going to evacuate anybody, either. People came here to be cared for, and that's what we are going to do."

"But we can't care for them very well if they aren't breathing. And what if the generators shut back down? Then we'll have two people without oxygen."

"I don't need the drama," she shot back. "The generators are not going to shut down. We have already dealt with that problem, and the maintenance man assures us they will continue running as long as we need them to."

I forced myself to look into her hard eyes and meet her steady gaze. "Can you be so sure of that?"

"Can you be so sure that they won't keep running? Come back when your man's oxygen tank runs out and then I'll ask the EMTs in the ambulance to loan us a tank."

"Can you ask them now, so I'll know they have one they can spare when this man's oxygen runs out?"

"I'm not going to wake them up. Check back later."

I went back to our room and related the conversation to Jan. We both felt like we were on the precipice of an impending doom and were helpless to do anything about it. We agreed that in a half-hour, we would call Alice, the Red Cross head nurse, and let her deal with McNutter.

A half-hour later, it happened. We heard the familiar thud, the lights blinked, then went off. We were in darkness again. We took the O2 saturation of both men on oxygen and were satisfied that both were in their mid 90s —for now.

While an oxygen tank has a volume of oxygen available in the tank, an oxygen concentrator does not. It uses the surrounding air to create an oxygen-rich mix, meaning the oxygen supply will never run out as long as the machine is powered and has access to an air supply. But if it has no power, it stops working and delivering oxygen to the patient.

I went back to find McNutter. She had a phone pressed to her ear.

"Pat, we need that oxygen tank now. Without power, our patient's oxygen concentrator is off."

"I'm too busy to deal with that right now. My priority is to get the power back on."

"My priority is to keep these men breathing. I'm going to ask the EMTs for that tank myself."

"You have no authority to ask them anything. I am in charge here and if there's going to be any asking, it will be by me, and I'm busy right now. The generator will kick back in in a few minutes just like it did before. Stop bothering me."

"And if it doesn't? Will you then transfer these patients out to the hospital?"

"Absolutely not."

I went back to monitor the two men. "She won't get the tank for us because she says she's too busy getting the generator to work. She still insists the generators will come back on. If Manny's oxygen gets close to 90%, we will have to put them both on the buddy system, using Joe's tank until I can get another tank over here."

We watched his POX drop to 93% in five minutes and then fall to 92% shortly after that. In fifteen minutes, he was at the critical 90% mark, and I could see that he was gasping more heavily for breath. I refused to let my thoughts dwell on what might happen.

"Put him on the buddy system with Joe's tank," I told Jan. "I'm going out to the ambulance for a tank."

I found Pat in a heated conversation with the maintenance man over the problems with the generator. He was telling her that some valve wasn't functioning and that he didn't have the part to fix it. She was insistent that he call someone else or find the part himself. In the middle of the argument, she looked up and saw me standing there.

"I'm getting that oxygen tank myself — now!" I yelled out to her as I turned away to find the EMTs.

Both of the EMT's were awake and emptying the rest of the coffee from the pot. I explained the situation and asked them for an oxygen tank. One said that they aren't authorized to loan out their supplies, but the other one said he would help. A few minutes later, he came back with a tank and handed it to me. I thanked him but as I was walking away, I looked down at the tank and realized there was no regulator gauge on the tank. Without it, I had no way to administer the oxygen. It was just a tank.

"Hey, guys. Do you have an oxygen regulator for this tank? I can't administer oxygen without it."

"We only have one," said the man who loaned me the tank. "We can't give you ours or we won't have it for our tank."

I walked back to the room and handed Jan the tank. "Do you want the good news or the bad news?" I asked her.

She looked up from the little POX indicator on Manny's finger. "Just start with the bad," she said in a monotone. "His POX is down to 89%."

"I have an oxygen tank but no gauge to administer oxygen."

"Then we have to get these guys out of here, now. Stay here and I'll go talk to McNutter."

I could see the anxiety and fear in Manny's eyes. "Am I going to be all right?" he asked, with a raspy cough.

"Of course," I said in my calm nurse's voice, but inside I was shaking. Then I realized that there was a gauge on Joe's tank. If I put that gauge on this new tank, then there would be enough oxygen to use the buddy system for a few more hours. I explained to them what I needed to do, and Joe handed me his tank.

I doubt that any nurse who worked less than thirty years as a nurse would know how to put a gauge on an oxygen tank. That job is now left to the respiratory therapists. All newer nurses are taught only how to link the nasal cannula up to the oxygen outlet that comes out of the wall. But forty years ago, I worked at the Martha's Vineyard cottage hospital. It only had twenty-five beds at the time. There was no air conditioning, but it really wasn't needed because the hospital was cleverly built so that when the windows were opened, the breeze off the Vineyard Sound would blow through the rooms on one side of the hallway straight over the ones to the other side. Both rooms were cooled with pure, clean ocean air. No one complained about being hot.

Nor did they have walled oxygen. When we needed oxygen, we called the maintenance man. He would wheel in a five-foot green tank and set it by the patient's bed. It was the nurse's job to "crack the tank," as they called it when we switched the gauge from one tank to another. There was a specific method for doing this. If you did it incorrectly, the oxygen blew out with a force that made it difficult to reset the gauge.

It had been thirty years since I cracked an oxygen tank and I had three sets of eyes watching me perform this task. I took a minute and went through the steps mentally and then prayed that I had it all right. I removed the nipple adaptor on the new tank, making sure the flow regulator was set at zero and that the T-bar or handle was tight. Then I placed the cylinder wrench on the on/off valve and set the amount of oxygen at one liter.

Administering oxygen to someone with emphysema can be tricky. For a patient with this disorder, or COPD as it is often called, the drive to breathe is reversed from normal people. When normal lungs are deprived of oxygen, the brain triggers that person to breathe deeper and more frequently to bring in more oxygen. However, too much oxygen for a COPDer can actually depress the patients' drive to breathe and they can stop breathing.

There are two different types of COPD. First, there are the "blue bloaters" with an illness is caused by chronic bronchitis. They are usually overweight and barrel-chested and have a chronic cough and audible wheeze. They often have a blue tinge around their lips and at the ends of their fingers. Manny was a "blue bloater."

The other type is the "pink puffer." Such patients are usually thin and breathe faster than normal breathers. Their faces develop a pink tinge as they struggle for a more effective air exchange. They tend to drop their POX quicker than the blue boaters. Joe was a "pink puffer."

I connected Joe to the spare tank first and then instructed him to switch over the oxygen cannula with Manny every three minutes, so that neither of them were without oxygen very long.

Chapter 10
"I'M SO COLD."

3:30am

"I'm so cold," came a weak voice from the corner of the room. It was my feeding tube woman. I was so concerned about finding oxygen for my two COPDers that I hadn't paid attention to the room temperature. Jan had a serious look on her face.

"When the power failed, the furnace also quit. We now have no heat."

The wind howled and whistled around the outside corner of our room, making it feel even colder. We gave each other that "now what?" look.

"I'll go out and try to find a warmer room," I told Jan. "Would you bring another blanket over to Mrs. LeBlanc and tell her we will try to find a warmer place?"

When I walked out into the hallway, I found it eerily quiet. The only sound was that of the wind wailing and slapping the snow against the windows. There was no one at the registration desk. "Where was Scott?" I wondered. Then I heard two people arguing in the communication room behind the desk.

"I don't know how long it will take," said a woman's voice.

"We had better damned well find out in a hurry, or we'll all freeze to death in here," said the man's voice that I now recognized as Scott's. "It looks like we may have to evacuate this shelter."

"I'm not going to let that happen. I'm in charge here and..." Pat swung around and glared at me as I entered the room.

I had picked up enough of the conversation to let them know that I had heard what was said. I noticed that the muscles in Scott's face tensed and the vein in his forehead was pounding.

"Scott is right. I have two patients with a limited amount of oxygen, a skeleton of a woman whose feeding tube isn't functioning and she is freezing cold, a woman who can't sleep without her CPAP machine, an elderly, obese woman who is in danger of falling off the exam table at any time and needs a physician to treat the cellulitis in her legs, and a diabetic for whom I had to scramble around to find food so his blood sugar wouldn't drop. If nothing shows up for breakfast any better than what we got for supper, he could go into a diabetic ketoacidosis."

I looked up to see Jan walk into the room.

"They are all okay for now," she assured me. She turned to McNutter. "I'm the head nurse for the Red Cross on the Cape. I know you are in charge here, but you aren't a medical professional. You have two nurses and an EMT standing in front of you telling you this situation is dire, especially now that we have no heat."

McNutter took on the commanding stance of an army drill sergeant about to address new recruits. "I know all of this. You are all overreacting. I've been told that they will get the generator running up within the hour, so go back to take care of your patients, and leave the running of this shelter up to me. It is my job." She emphasized the word "my."

"You had better have it running up within the hour," I replied. "Because that dinky little oxygen tank I got from the ambulance won't last much longer than maybe two hours. Do you want to be responsible if these two men go into respiratory arrest?"

She took one hand off her hip and pointed to Jan and me. "That's your jobs. Not mine."

She turned her back and picked up the phone, indicating that this conversation was over. I stood there frozen, staring at her back. I felt powerless. The ability to keeping my patients safe seemed to slide away beneath me. I felt like I was the chief mate on a ship in the middle a storm staring into a giant wave that the captain ignored.

I tried to regain some sense of restraint. I paused for a moment to regain my thoughts and turning to Scott, I tried to sound like I was in control. "Scott, I can't get these patients moved out..." I cleared my throat. "...but we can at least try to make them more comfortable while they are here. Is there a warmer room to move these people to? I've got a woman who is barely 90 pounds, an elderly woman, a ten-year-old boy, a woman on chemo, and a few others. I need to be able to keep them warmer. Do you have any suggestions?"

"Let me look around." He put his hand on my shoulder in the gesture of a big brother assuring his kid sister. "Look, I'm on your side. I'll let you know if I hear anything about the generator or find a warmer room. Thanks for everything you both are doing. I know this isn't easy."

We went back and looked around at the solemn faces of our patients who knew that all was not going well. I announced to everyone that we were looking for a warmer room, then spoke to each of them individually as I handed out blankets.

"Don't worry, Max. We'll keep an eye on your blood sugar."

I tousled Jack's hair. "I'm so proud of how you care for your mom."

I put my hand on the boney shoulder of Mrs. LeBlanc. "You'll be more comfortable in a warmer room."

I took Jan aside. "Have you ever been in this situation before?" I asked her as she came toward me with an armful of blankets.

"No. And I can assure you I will discuss this at the monthly meeting so it doesn't happen again."

"So how did this Pat McNutter get to be a shelter manager? I mean what organization sponsors her?"

"None that I know of. It's most likely a political placement."

"Political? And she has the right to refuse medical professionals' advice?"

"Unfortunately, yes."

As we were handing out the blankets, Scott came to the door. "I found a room that is just above the furnace. It has retained some of the heat. It's just down the hall. I'll help you move people over there."

The floor creaked as we wheeled Manny, Joe, and Mrs. LeBlanc in wheelchairs down to the room. The air in it was like an old attic that hadn't been opened in years, but I welcomed the warmth. I could feel the difference in my hands.

For years I have dealt with Raynaud's Syndrome in both hands. It makes my hands react abnormally to the cold. First my fingers turn red, then blue, and then white. When they turn white, I lose all feeling in them and have to work quickly to warm them up and return them to a normal color. Delay could cause ulceration in my fingertips. I often joked that I have patriotic fingertips.

I keep little disposable hot packs with me in the winter because gloves are never enough. Now I took two of them out, activated them by shaking them, and put them in my pockets, where I could close my hands around them. As my hands absorbed the warmth, they began to ache. It took a while for the feeling to return, but gradually they turned back to a normal color.

The exam table was on wheels, so while carefully guarding the sides, we wheeled our 90-year-old over with the others. The group had now formed a camaraderie with each other. Joe shared his magazines, Cathy, the pica woman, shared some of her treasured food items, and the MS lady began to break out in familiar songs. *"Oh, the weather outside is frightful. But the fire is so delight-ful."*

Soon they all joined in singing with her as they huddled in their blankets. I was able to keep Manny's and Joe's POX above 90% by switching the oxygen tank back and forth between them, but I knew this tank would barely last until the morning. What then?

113

Chapter 11
PLAN B DENIED

4:30am

Jan and I gave up trying to sleep. Another hour went by, and still the generators did not start up. I could feel the heat slowly seeping out of the room. I checked the oxygen tank. We had enough oxygen for about two hours. "We are playing Russian roulette with these patients," I said to Jan.

"There has to be a way to move them out. Betty is still on call for Alice, the Red Cross chief nurse. I'm calling Betty once more and then Alice. Hell, we're not sleeping. Why should they?" I smiled.

Jan handed me her phone and I called Betty first. It rang until the answering machine picked up. I left another message.

Then I called Alice. My heart jumped when I heard her voice. "Alice, we have a situation here you need to know about. We need your help. Betty hasn't been answering her phone, and I didn't want to call you, but I have to now." I explained what was happening.

"And the generator hasn't gone on?"

"No, and that was more than an hour ago. It goes on for while, and then it keeps going off, but this time, it hasn't come back on. I've got about two hours left on the borrowed tank that these two COPDers are sharing. Then, I have no Plan B other than to send them both to the hospital or a local rehab facility or a nursing home—somewhere that can meet their needs."

"Put me on the phone with Pat McNutter," Alice said.

Jan was watching me for a positive sign of cooperation. When I gave her a thumbs-up, she returned the gesture. "Stay on the line, Alice, and I'll put you on speaker, and we'll have that conversation together."

"Wait!" said Alice. "Is it even possible to transport people in the middle of this storm in the middle of the night?"

"Good question. Let me talk to Scott. He's the EMT in charge of the registration desk. Everyone congregates around that desk, so he is in the middle of the action. I'll call you back."

Jan went back to check on our patients, including the man with the flu. We bundled him up in blankets until we could find a warmer room for him. I couldn't put him in the same room as the others. He too needed to be evacuated.

I found Scott in the staff room discussing the storm with the ambulance driver, another EMT, and a man I didn't know. "Scott, is it possible to get my patients out of here to a facility that can handle their needs?" He thought for a moment and then turned to address the staff he was just talking to. "So do any of you know if it is possible to transfer some of these people out?"

The ambulance driver was the first to respond. "If we can get them to send in a plow that can open us up here and plow ahead of us, I think we can do it."

The other EMT joined in. "None of these people have a problem that can't be solved by being in the right place. That doesn't have to be the hospital ER. The rehab hospital is a lot closer. Maybe they would be willing to take them for the next day or so."

The man I didn't know pulled out a communications device that looked like a short-wave radio. "I can call them right now and see what they'll say. Give me a minute." We all stood by listening to the conversation. "Yes, there are..." He cupped his hand over the phone. "How many people do you want sent out?"

"At least 5."

He uncupped his hand. "Five patients. Two with COPD — oxygen dependent, one frail woman with a feeding pump, one woman on a CPAP machine, and a 92-year-old with multiple care issues. The nurses here are Terri Arthur and ..."

"Jan Holloway."

"Jan Holloway. Terri is the Red Cross nurse and Jan is the head nurse of the MRC. Okay. Thanks, I'll tell them."

Jan had just walked into the room. He addressed us both. "They said they'll take the two COPDers and the feeding pump lady but not the other two. I'm in charge of communications so if you want me to call for that plow..."

"Thanks..." I looked at his name tag. "... Rob." We have to talk this over with McNutter first."

"You won't find her in the communications room. She's downstairs with the maintenance guy trying to get the generator to kick back in. Do you want me to call her to talk to us?"

"Tell her we'll meet her at the admissions table."

We both felt some relief that there was a safe resource for the most needy of our patients. At least now we could discuss an option with McNutter. Jan, Scott, I, and the other staff members waited about fifteen minutes before she came walking down the hall towards us. I called Alice back and put the phone on speaker.

"Pat, we have a very unsafe situation here. I have Alice Kent-Levinson on the phone to join in on this conversation. Do you know who she is?"

"No, who's she?"

"She's the chief nurse of the Red Cross on the Cape. The other nurse with me is Jan Holloway who is the head nurse of the MRC.

Scott is an EMT. In addition, we have an ambulance driver here and the communications director. I've explained our dilemma to them. Alice agrees that these patients must be sent to a safer facility, and the others here are an ambulance driver, and two EMTs. We have an idea as to how to do it."

Pat crossed her arms across her chest. "Not going to happen. I've been working with the maintenance man to get the generator fixed, and we're expecting it will be back on track as soon as he replaces a part."

Scott joined in. "Look Pat. We, and by that, I mean all of us here, including you, aren't going to look very good if these patients get sicker on our watch. The missing part has to be found before it can be replaced, so we really have no idea how long this generator will be off."

Alice's voice came from the phone speaker. "In the meantime, we are responsible for these people. I understand that the rehab center down the road is willing to take the patients we're most concerned about."

I joined in. "And Rob is checking right now to see if he can get a plow here to dig us out and clear the way ahead of the ambulance."

McNutter gave each of us an icy stare. "And you did this without checking with me first?"

I jumped in. "We're checking with you now. Rob will let you know when the plow can arrive here."

"You had no right to make that decision without my permission."

It was Jan's turn. "Pat, you have three nurses, an EMT—two actually, including the ambulance driver—standing here telling you that these patients need to go somewhere else to be kept safe. They are not safe here. Why won't you work with us to move them to a place that can better serve their needs?"

"Because I'm in charge here, not any of you. I am responsible for everyone who comes to this shelter. They will be staying here until someone comes to pick them up or they leave on their own and from the looks of this storm that isn't going to happen for at least another day. The generator should be up and running soon."

"And if it isn't?" asked Scott.

"Then we'll talk about some other plan. Maybe we'll send them to another shelter that still has power."

The three of us walked away, with Alice still on connected on the phone in my hand. "So what do you think, Alice?" I asked her.

"Maybe she's right. Maybe we should send them to another shelter."

"I have no problem with that. But the problem is, how long do we wait? We have enough oxygen for about two hours. Do we really want to wait that long?"

"I can check with the closest shelter and get back to you."

Jan's patience ran out. "Scott, stay here. I'm calling up the head of the Cape's Coalition of Emergency Services (CCES). He's the big honcho. We'll get Alice on the line as well. McNutter is responsible to him. And I think he will agree with five medical people who are advising him that something has to be done. He won't want dead bodies on his hands."

Chapter 12
STAN LAWRENCE

5:00am

Jan had the head of the CCES on speed dial. "Hey, Stan. It's Jan Holloway of the MRC. I'm sorry to be calling you so early, but we have an emergency situation here at the Shelton shelter and we need you to help us work it through."

"No problem, Jan. I'm not sleeping anyway. Too much going on tonight. What's up?"

Jan explained our predicament, ending up with, "We can't get Pat McNutter to agree to evacuate some of these people, especially the ones who need oxygen. They are on borrowed time as the oxygen in the one tank they are sharing is about to run out."

"Pat who?"

"Pat McNutter. The shelter manager."

"Who in God's name is she? I've never heard of her."

"Well she's here all right, and she's running the show. The power is off and the back-up generator won't start. There is no heat, and everyone is huddled up in army blankets. She refuses to evacuate anyone because she insists the generator will come back on."

"And will it? Come back on, that is?"

"It came back on twice but has been off for an hour now. They need a part to make it work and don't have it."

"Put McNutter on the phone. Put it on speaker and hand it to her." We walked back to where Jan was standing and handed the phone over to Pat with a brief introduction. "This is Stan Lawrence. He's the head of the Cape's Coalition of Emergency Services."

Pat looked at Jan and then back at me. She flipped her hair away from both ears, hesitated and then said, "This is Pat McNutter."

"Ms. McNutter, you have sick people in your charge. We need to find a way for them to be evacuated. What plans have you made to do so?

McNutter's lips tightened. "Mr. Lawrence, I was told that I needed to be responsible for everyone who comes to this shelter, and I take that responsibility very seriously."

His voice was hard as granite. "Well, here's the bottom line, Ms. McNutter. I take my responsibility seriously too, and I don't like hearing that there are people in our shelters who might get sicker and even die because we didn't do everything we could to make them safe. Do you understand?"

McNutter nervously shifted her weight from one foot to the other and glared at everyone standing around her. She lowered her voice.

"Yes, sir."

"Jan tells me that there is barely and hour or two left of oxygen for these two people who are dependent on it...."

"Yes, but..."

"I'm not through talking!" His voice cut through the air like a bullet and landed like a mortar. "I understand there's a woman who needs a machine to breathe at night."

Pat took on an expression that was somewhere between irritation and intimidation. "Well, yes, but..."

"Don't interrupt me!...and there's a woman who has been off her feeding tube for over five hours. Is this true?"

"The nurses mentioned that to me."

"And for as long as an hour each time the electricity is out, the heating system cannot supply heat."

"But what can I do in this storm? There's a plow in the driveway that broke down under the weight of the snow and..."

"Then you call me. You do know who I am, don't you?"

"I've heard your name mentioned."

"I don't know who you are, but I'm going to find out who you are and how you got to be put in this position. But for now, I am going to call in a heavy-duty plow to clean out your driveway. I will then have it plow in front of the ambulance to clear the roads for them. I want those people with medical needs out as soon as the plow arrives.

"As for the rest of the people you have there, remove the four who are under medical care first, and then evacuate the other four to nearby shelters. I'll call the other shelters and see how many more people they can take in. Then I'll get back to you. Do you understand?"

"Yes, Mr. Lawrence. But what if the generator comes back on?"

"Enough about the God-damned generator that is unreliable. Move those people out to a safe place, whether it's the hospital or another shelter."

"Yes, sir." McNutter clicked the phone off and handed it back to Jan. I looked over to Scott and saw a faint smile hover over his lips. Jan's eyes locked onto McNutter's, waiting for her next move. Trying to take in what had just happened, McNutter looked around at everyone standing around her. She ran the tip of her tongue over her lips, then cleared her throat. "Looks like we have some work to do."

She turned away from Jan and addressed the ambulance EMT. "You said that the rehab hospital is willing to take the two men on oxygen?" He nodded a yes. "Call them back and tell them that we will be transferring them over to their care as soon as the plow cleans out the driveway."

Then she turned to Jan and me. "Which of the other ones should be sent to the hospital?"

I felt myself exhale a breath that I hadn't realized I was holding. Finally we were addressing the medical needs of these patients. "Definitely the elderly woman with the infected legs and the woman on the feeding pump. The one on the CPAP machine can go to another shelter as long as they have power. The others can go there too. We do have one man with the flu."

I turned to the ambulance EMT. "Do you have a spare mask?"

"I'm sure I do."

"It's five o'clock now. Sunrise is around seven. It will probably take about that long to get the plow here and have the driveway plowed out."

Then I asked the EMT. "You have one more oxygen tank in your ambulance, right?" He nodded in agreement. "Good; then, if we can't transfer our COPD patients out before their oxygen runs out, and you can't hand over your last oxygen tank, we'll have to put them in the ambulance and have them share your tank with the buddy system."

Jan and I discussed how we would prioritize our patients for transfer and then headed back to the room where we explained the plan to everyone. I addressed the worried faces. "I know it will get colder while we are waiting to leave, so tell me if any of you need more blankets. We do have plenty of those."

"How about a hot cup of coffee?" asked the man with the cast on his leg.

"Don't I wish," said Jan.

"How about a candy bar or chocolate?" asked Joe.

"Got a sweet tooth?" I joked.

"No. I just took my blood sugar and it's 80. I didn't eat much supper.

Normal blood sugar levels range from 80 to 120, although the results vary from lab to lab. Joe's level was borderline but could drop dangerously, causing hypoglycemia. That could cause dizziness, lack of coordination, change in mentation, sweating, and even death, if untreated.

I knew exactly where to find the sugar he needed. I took out the three chocolate chip cookies that I had brought from home and went over to Cathy's cot. She was sitting up, eating Doritos out of a bag. "Cathy, do you want some more chocolate chip cookies?"

"Do you have some?"

"I do, but I need to know if you have any chocolate or candy bars in your food bag."

She fished around in her cloth bag and came up with a Mounds bar.

"Can I trade these homemade cookies for that Mounds bar?" I asked.

"How many cookies?"

"Three."

"I'll do it for four."

"I only have three. What if I throw in a pack of Oreo cookies. Will that do?"

She agreed to the trade and gave me the Mounds bar. I asked Jan to go down to the cafeteria to see if any of the cookies Donna had been giving out were still available. There was only one pack of Oreos left that Donna had saved for herself, but she handed it over to Jan. I gave the Oreo package to Cathy and the Mounds bar to Joe.

"Keep track of your blood sugar, so we can keep you within normal range." With a mouth full of chocolate and coconut, he agreed.

Manny eyed his oxygen buddy's candy with a bit of envy. "Jeez. You got another one of those around? I didn't get much to eat either." I promised him I would look around and get back to him. More bargaining with Cathy produced a NutButter bar, which I handed over to Manny.

An hour later, I heard the motor and rough scraping noise of a plow outside. I wasn't surprised at how long it took him to get here because there was a long side road to the

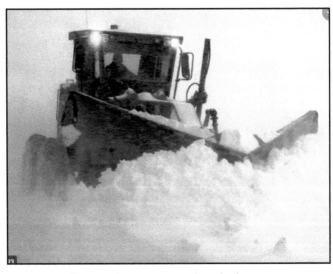

Snow plow sent to the shelter.
(Photo by Terri Arthur)

130

high school. That meant he had to plow that out before he got to the circular driveway outside the school. It took him another half-hour to plow out the driveway.

When the driver came through the door, he looked like a refugee from the Gulag. He stamped the snow off his boots, threw his coat hood back, and removed his thick gloves.

He told Scott, "I can't plow around that plow that's stuck in the driveway. There are cars parked on each side of it. If you have the keys, I'll try to come around on the other side and plow in front of it, and then I might be able to move it out of the driveway. But to do that, a few feet of snow has to be shoveled out. Can you help me out with that?"

Scott called for a couple of the Ameri-Corps kids to come up and help shovel out the plow. It wouldn't be an easy thing to do in the dark with the air still thick with snow and the wind like needles stinging their faces.

My heart sank when I heard about the delay. Jan had been carefully watching the oxygen tank level. We both knew it was already dangerously low.

"We need to go to plan B, or is it plan C? We've had so many plans, I lost track," said Jan.

"That may be true. But the plan you had to call the head of the CCES was brilliant! Aren't you full of surprises?"

"Desperate times, call for desperate measures."

Twenty minutes later, the plow driver reappeared at the reception desk. "You're all plowed out for now. I'll try to start the plow that's stuck in the driveway and run it up the sidewalk or on the lawn or at least where we think the lawn and sidewalk would be if they weren't under two feet of snow. We have to move quickly or the wind will blow every-thing back over it."

I found the two ambulance EMTs at the reception desk talking to Scott and joined their conversation. "The two COPDers are running out of oxygen. I need to move them to your ambulance. One of you will have to stay with them until you can get moving."

I heard the engine of the stuck plow turn over and then stop and start several times. The plow driver came back in announcing, "Can't get the damn thing to start. I'll have to plow a path over on the grassy area around the cars and then we can get started. He turned to the two EMTs. "You two ready?"

"As soon as we move the two patients into the ambulance," they answered.

We wrapped the two men up in blankets and put them both in wheelchairs to make the move easier for them. The AmeriCorps kids shoveled a walkway from the school door to the ambulance, but it was too narrow for wheelchairs, so Manny and Joe were slowly assisted by the EMTs down the narrow path and into the ambulance.

I felt a wave of relief when I saw them through the open doors of the ambulance, attach Joe's nasal cannula up to their tank. Manny was using the last of what was left in the loaned tank. They waved back at Jan and me just before the EMTs closed the doors.

We stood inside the doorway watching the slow procession of plow and ambulance clear the driveway and head down the road to the rehabilitation center. Two down and three more to go, plus the others who had been admitted into our medical care. It would be daylight soon. That would make the other transfers easier.

Chapter 13
SLEEP DEPRIVATION

7:00am

Once I saw my two most worrisome patients leave for safety, I felt a sudden weariness. I hadn't slept for 22 hours. "Interesting," I thought. "The last time I went without sleep this long was also during a snowstorm."

I had been working the evening shift at Cape Cod Hospital on a 30-bed orthopedic unit. The nurse/patient ratio was 1:5 but we also had to cover the LPNs for orders and IV medications, and of course, everything that was medical for the patients that were assigned to the aides. So often the RN really had fifteen patients if she worked with a LPN and an aide.

Frequently, the weather from Falmouth, where I lived, was quite different from that of Hyannis, seventeen miles from where the hospital was located. I could leave Falmouth with the sun shining and arrive in Hyannis in a torrential rainstorm.

On that particular evening, I had left Falmouth on a sunny winter day and arrived in Hyannis during a raging snowstorm. As the evening went on, I hoped the snow would subside, but it didn't. At the end of my shift, the night staff couldn't make it in. There was no one to relieve us. I couldn't walk out, and even if I were able to, the snow had piled high enough that I couldn't drive home.

One nurse, a big Irish woman named Mary O'Brien, said she could make it home because she had a Jeep with four-wheel drive. Since the night shift normally had one less nurse, she was allowed to leave.

The storm continued throughout the night. A few hours into the night shift, I felt that my eyes were stinging and irritated as I read the medication sheets. Digoxin, a cardiac med, began to look like Doxipen, a sleeping medication. I had to check and recheck to be sure I was giving out the right med.

Finally the morning came, and having been awake now for 23 hours, I could barely concentrate. My legs felt stiff and heavy. I was eager to see the day shift staff come in and take over. But the day staff didn't come in, because they couldn't make it through the piles of snow.

Breakfast trays were brought up for us to hand out, and many patients required someone to feed them. I had a mid-morning med pass to hand out medications, and there were frequent requests for pain medication. There was no one to answer the phones. I ran from patient to medication cart to the phone and back again. My scrubs were wrinkled, and I could smell the sweat running down my sides. My whole body ached.

I was at the desk answering the phone when two supervisors appeared. Both were in their pressed street clothes, low heels, flawless make-up, and sporting crisp white lab coats with their names neatly embroidered on their left shoulder. Each cradled a clipboard in her arm.

"We're here to help you," chirped one of them, flashing a Colgate smile. The other one flipped a paper on her clipboard. "You are...?"

"Terri Arthur. I'm one of the evening nurses, and I'm dragging it, so I welcome whatever help you both can give us."

"Could you..." I pointed to the Colgate supervisor, "start at the beginning of the unit and help feed patients and set people up to be washed? And you..." I said, pointing to the clipboard holder, "could you please start passing out medications on the other side?"

"Oh, I'm sorry," said the Colgate supervisor. I don't do patient care."

"And I don't give out medications on patients I don't know," said the clipboard holder."

I stood stunned. "What do you both do?"

"We can answer the phones," said the clipboard holder.

"Oh, good, really good. Then how about if you..." addressing Ms. Colgate, "sit over there, get on the phone, and find some nurses who actually do patient care."

I turned to Ms. Clipboard. "And you could get on the other phone and find some nurses who give out medications."

They seemed excited. "We'll try! Anything to help out," they chirped.

I barely remember what happened the rest of the day shift. I think they sent over a maternity nurse, who announced when she arrived that she couldn't have an assignment in case she had to be called back to the maternity unit. It was all a blur. I felt drugged or at least suffering from a bad hangover. I could feel myself moving in slow motion and not getting medications out on time.

I knew I was unsafe — very unfit to care for patients. I remember losing my spatial ability. I think that's what you call it when you lose the capacity to judge the relation of one object to another. For instance, I would misjudge how much water to pour into a glass and fill it until it overflowed or offer a patient a medication and miss putting it their hand.

An hour before the day shift was over, the only thing I do remember was the sight of Mary O'Brien striding down the hallway in her L.L. Bean boots and a puffy big, blue, full-length coat. She had a large cup of Dunkin' Donuts coffee in one hand and in the other a L.L. Bean canvas boat bag with her initials embroidered on the side. She was her usual bouncy self.

"You look like hell," she greeted me as she handed me the cup of coffee.

"And you look like an angel," I answered, taking the coffee and sipping it. "Gawd, this tastes good! How are the roads?"

"Terrible. I don't think I could have made it in without the Jeep. They are just now plowing the roads clean, so they should be better when you leave. Where is everybody?"

"Everybody? Ha! You're it!" As the hours passed, the evening shift staff began to trickle in. I had been awake for 30 hours before I left, and I still had to dig my car out of a snowbank and drive home on dangerously slippery roads.

I remember gripping the steering wheel, turning the volume up on the radio, and cracking the window open so the cold air would keep me awake. What I remember most about that experience was how disoriented I felt. I imagined that this must be what it felt like to be on some kind of hallucinogenic drug. I guess the simple word for it was "zoned out."

It had only been 24 hours since I hadn't slept but that was how I was starting to feel now. Remembering that past experience, I knew why I was feeling like I had a hangover. I could pull myself together, but I wasn't on top of my game. My eyes began to sting and my steps felt leaden. I forced myself to focus.

One of the volunteers walked by with a cup of coffee. "Hey! Where did you get that?" I asked.

"A policeman brought in a cup 'o joe from Dunkin' Donuts. It's in a little cove on the left about twenty feet down the hall. It's not very hot any more."

"All I care is if it has caffeine in it," I called back as I headed down the hall.

Chapter 14
FOOD FOR THOUGHT

8:05am

It was now past 8:00am and no food had arrived. We were all getting hungry and hoped breakfast would be coming soon. Scott's short-wave radio kept us up to date on what was happening in the outside world.

> *The Cape has taken a hit as this massive storm hammers the area with wind and snow. The National Grid said it would take longer than first thought to restore power. NStar indicated that some of its customers might not have power for three days. Both utilities said their power delivery systems sustained heavy damage. The crews continue to struggle with impassable roads and deep snow blocking access to equipment. New outages continue to occur, caused by snow and ice-laden tree limbs snapping out power lines.*

I went downstairs to find out from Donna what was holding up breakfast. My woman with the tube feeding had not received any nourishment for about eight hours. Jack, the ten-year-old, kept coming up to the desk and asking when breakfast would arrive. His mother tried to console him but I knew she was also hungry. The banana I had given her and the cookies for the boy last night were no where near enough to satisfy either of them.

The only one who was satisfied was Cathy, our pica woman, who had brought a knapsack of food. I was sure she wouldn't part with it if I didn't have anything to trade with her. Everyone was commenting about the cold. I could see that Mrs. LeBlanc, my frail feeding-tube woman, was shivering under the layers of blankets I had piled around her.

Donna was sitting in the cafeteria staring out a wall of windows at the raging storm. I sat next to her. "If there's food in this kitchen, Donna, we need to give it out to the people here. We can deal with the consequences later on."

"There's over 50 people here besides your eight. We'll never find enough to feed all of them. How do we dole it out? Next thing you know, we'll have a riot. And besides, I don't know where there is any food."

We stood at the door of the kitchen and looked into the vast land of steel counters, deep soapstone sinks, monolithic steel refrigerators with locks on their doors, and white enamel cabinets lined along the walls. There were side rooms off the main kitchen. Donna turned to me. "I wouldn't know where to start trying to find anything in here."

"Well, guess what?" I smiled. "I know someone who does know exactly where we could find something to eat. I'll be back."

In a few minutes, I returned with Cathy, the pica lady, in tow. She was spooning pudding out of a plastic cup.

"Cathy, can you show us where you found the cereal, milk, and yogurt yesterday evening?"

"I think so. It looks so different today but..." She walked over to what looked like locked refrigerators. "I got milk and yogurt out of here," and opened the door to one of them.

"But there are locks on those doors. How did you open them?"

"The locks aren't really locked. See?" She twisted open the stem on one of the locks.

"And the cereal boxes. Where were those?"

She walked into a side room to the right of the kitchen. "The cabinets in here have cereal boxes in them." Then she started to get excited. "There were cardboard boxes somewhere piled up that had cookies and chips in them. I almost got a bunch of those until you caught me and made me stop."

Donna and I looked at each other. I put my hand over my mouth to keep from laughing. We found the boxes piled up against the back wall and opened them up. She was right. One had little packages of cookies, and the other had various bags of potato chips, Cheetos, potato sticks, and popcorn.

Donna took the cookies and chips up to the people who weren't sick, and I took the milk, cereal, and yogurt up to my patients. I also threw in a few packs of cookies for Jack. Jan and I each had a yogurt. Betty said she could drink some of the milk if she did it slowly. Jack's mother said the yogurt would help until food arrived, and Jack was quite happy to

have cereal with milk and cookies for breakfast. It was around 10:00 when McNutter
appeared at the door.

Her voice was subdued. "We are starting
to evacuate people to other shelters, so bring
your people out to the lobby by the reception
table. We'll be able to take three people at a
time depending on whether they are in a
wheelchair or have special needs. Then only
two will fit in the ambulance."

Jan and I began to bring our patients out
into the lobby two at a time. The lobby was
even colder than the room we had been in.
Every time the door was opened, a swirl of
snow and frigid air blew inside, making the
entrance wet and slippery. First, McNutter
took the self-care patient who was on chemo
and the man on crutches with the torn
Achilles repair.

Jan and I looked at each other and stepped
aside to discuss our concerns. "Shouldn't the
92-year-old and the woman on the feeding
tube be going first?" Jan asked me.

"She didn't ask me who should go first or
last," I said as I shoved my hands into my
pockets to keep them warm. We both walked
over to McNutter. "Can we talk to you?"

McNutter turned her back to us as she checked off a clipboard of people's names. "Yes, make it quick. I'm busy sending these people to another shelter."

I walked around to face her. "Why are the two patients with the least serious problems going first? It should be the ones who have the most needs."

Pat took that familiar military stance with her hands across her chest. We knew what that meant, and she didn't disappoint our expectations. "I am still in charge here and I will determine who leaves first."

Just then, we heard a thud and a whirr and the lights went on. The generator had started back up.

"See?" she threw out at us. "I told you the generator would go back on. Now all of this is a waste of time and staff."

"Pat, that may be so, but we still don't know how long it will stay on. We need to stop taking chances with this generator and just move these people to safer places."

Pat turned and walked away.

We found an outlet for the feeding pump to work; then I took the woman aside and asked her to flush her own stomach tube. She fumbled a bit but was successful. I gave her a little hug and told her how proud I was of her. She beamed with pride. "My daughter is going to be so happy that she won't have to keep coming to my house to do this."

A half hour later, the ambulance returned. One of the EMTs carried a bag in with him. He walked over to the registration desk and dumped about a dozen sandwiches onto the desk.

"This was all we could scrounge up for food," he announced. Immediately staff members snatched up the sandwiches before the people could reach them. I was amazed at the brazen behavior of the staff, but I knew how they felt. I had given my last banana to the woman with MS and my peanut butter cookies to her son. I shared one of the two pre-packaged cups of dry oatmeal with Jan. We moistened them with water. We gave out the remaining yogurts and the few remaining cookies to everyone else.

I hadn't slept in 25 hours. My whole body was weary and screamed at me to lie down and take a nap. My eyes watered with the burning.

I squeezed them shut and opened them again to stop the discomfort. It didn't work. I offered a silent plea. "Please, eyes, don't fail me now." Jan looked as weary as I felt. I suggested that she go back and try to take a catnap.

"Thanks," she said, rubbing her red-lined eyes. "But if I lie down now, you won't be able to wake me up. Besides, we still have to help transfer these patients out."

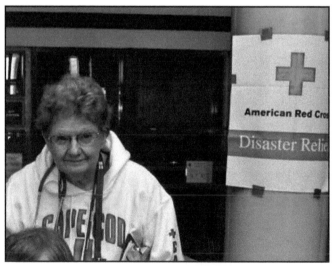

The author wheeling out Mrs. LeBlanc, to be transferred to another shelter.

Chapter 15

THE LAST TRANSFER

Over the next two hours, McNutter orchestrated the gradual transportation of our patients to a shelter in Falmouth. The only one left was the man with the flu. Just as the woman who was on chemo was being assisted into the ambulance, I saw Scott bring someone over to the registration desk. The person he was signing in was a very obese woman in a wide-body wheelchair. The nasal cannula on her face snaked down to an oxygen tank strapped to the side of the wheelchair.

Pushing the wheelchair was a younger man who, I soon found out, had a mental disability. I heard her say she was a diabetic and needed to have her blood sugar checked.

Scott handed me her admission sheet:

> Name: Sally Duggan, 56
> Son: Nathan, 31
>
> Problem: COPD, oxygen dependent, diabetic, and incontinent. Wheelchair

dependent due to obesity. Only able to walk short distances with assistance.

Additional: Son Nathan is mentally disabled and totally dependent on his mother.

"Scott, can I talk to you—alone?"

"In the communication room," he gestured.

"Why are you admitting this patient?"

"Because McNutter said to admit her."

"But we are evacuating all of the patients. Why would we admit someone who is in worse shape than the ones we just moved out? Why not just bring her over to the other shelter for them to admit her?"

"Ask McNutter."

"Could you please bring her back here for us to talk about this? I'm going to get Jan."

McNutter arrived in the communications room just as I appeared with Jan. She had a cup of coffee in one hand and the other dug into her pocket. She did the usual sassy hair flip before speaking. "What is it now?"

"Why are you admitting this woman when we are evacuating all our patients to another shelter? Just send her out with the others and let the other shelter admit her."

McNutter took a sip of her coffee and addressed us over the edge of the cup. "She came here for help, and that's what we are doing. The back-up generators are working."

"But that makes no sense. She's stable and we are just going to have to turn her around and move her out."

"I'm still in charge here, and if I say she needs to be admitted, then we admit her until I decide when to transfer her."

Just then, the son of the wheelchair-bound woman, came to the door. "My mother needs to go to the bathroom. She needs to have her pad changed too."

Jan and I stood stunned and couldn't move for a moment. Neither of us had to say anything. We were both tired and emotionally weary.

After we toileted her and cleaned her up, we took her blood sugar. It was 88. Neither she nor her son had eaten since last night. Jan went back to the room to find anything that was left over from what we had brought up from the kitchen earlier. Nothing was left, so I went back to the kitchen and retraced Cathy's steps from the refrigerator to the back cabinets to the boxes of cookies and was able to retrieve a small bag of peanuts, two boxes of cereal, and two containers of milk.

"That's all there is to eat around here?" asked the woman. "Nathan is hungry."

Jan jumped in. "I'm sorry, but I'm afraid we've been short on food here, and what little we had is gone. You will soon be transferred to a facility that will be better able to feed you and your son."

The woman tore open the bag of peanuts. "I hope it's soon. This is ridiculous."

Nathan was anxious about being in an unfamiliar place. He followed us around with various requests — he asked for water, needed to go to the bathroom, wanted more cookies, asked for a toothbrush, and a comb for his hair, and his dry socks because his were wet.

After all of my other patients had been transferred, McNutter finally transferred the wheelchair-bound woman and her son. They were the last of my patients to leave.

In the next few hours, McNutter worked to transfer out the rest of the people who had come to the shelter.

Chapter 16
GOING HOME

12:00noon

Now that all of the shelter people were gone, the staff scurried about breaking things down, bringing supplies back to the storage room downstairs, and packing up equipment that had to be transferred out. It was like looking at the movie of our set-up yesterday — in reverse.

Jan and I repacked our tubs and made a list of the supplies that needed to be replaced. We taped the tubs back up with adhesive tape and took the lists with us to bring back to our Red Cross headquarters for restocking. We were almost too tired to talk. Neither of us had slept for 28 hours. Jan loaned me her phone so I could let my sister and Elaine know that I'd be coming home soon.

"How are you going to get home?" asked Elaine. "It's still snowing and nothing has been plowed."

"Maybe the main roads will be plowed by the time I get there. You'll have a bone-weary and hungry girl on your hands."

"You've got a hot cup of coffee, a hot meal, and a hot woman waiting for you. Just get here safe and I'll take care of the rest."

I listened to the TV in the hallway as I stuffed my personal belongings back into my canvas boat bag.

> *Waves off the South Shore of Boston and parts of Cape Cod measured as high as 20 feet. The National Weather Service received reports of flooding up and down the Massachusetts coast, especially in areas just north and south of Boston. Water carrying slabs of ice sloshed through the streets and lapped against houses. Estimates are that the bluffs at Cape Cod National Seashore have lost 10-20 feet, exposing an ancient cedar swamp.*

> *In Connecticut an 81-year-old woman using a snow blower was hit by a car, a man in Bridgeport was found dead under*

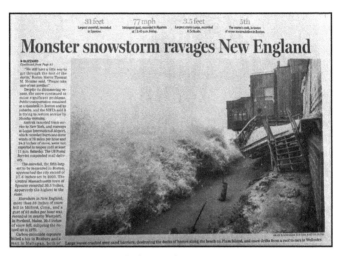

Boston Globe, February 10, 2013

the snow at his home, and a man died
after he suffered a heart attack while
plowing snow in New Milford. In Shelton a
man died while...

I looked up to see Jan standing in front of me. "My husband's coming to pick me up. He said they are starting to plow the main roads. He has a big ole four-wheel-drive Jeep Wrangler, so if we go slow, I should be able to get home safely. How are you getting home?"

"I'll have to dig my car out. It's an SUV Toyota Rav 4 and has a four-wheel drive, so I should be okay."

156

I gave her a hug. "Hey, you were amazing. I couldn't have done this gig without you. Let's keep in touch. And about McNutter, I'm going to find out who in the hell she is."

"I'll ask around too. You take care." Jan turned to go out the door and then turned back. "You know, I'm always looking for good nurses to work with me in the Medical Corps. So any time you get tired of working for the Red Cross, or you want a change..."

"Thanks. I'm sticking with the Red Cross for now, but I'll keep your offer in mind."

I pulled on my boots, tied a woolen scarf around my neck, and zipped up my L.L. Bean ultra-warm Maine winter jacket. I stuffed two heating pads into my gloves, flipped my faux-fur hood over my head, shouldered my bag, and headed for the door. The registration desk had already been cleared of papers, phones, and clipboards. I looked around for Scott but didn't see him.

I stood staring out the front glass doors and hesitated. It was still snowing and the wind swirled into a break-dance around the mounds of snow. I shuddered but went through the doors to where I hoped my car was parked.

I could feel the fingers of frigid air creeping down my neck. The snow crunched under my boots as I walked. I felt the cold melting down into my socks and into my boots. This would be a problem if I couldn't get out of the cold. The wetness would freeze my toes, aggravating the Reynaud's in my feet. My face stung as the snow pelted it. I felt my cheeks flush in response to the new onslaught of cold.

When I reached my car, the only thing visible was the antenna. I brushed off enough of the snow to get to the door handle. The shovel and ice scraper were inside. I chastised myself for not thinking what a foolish idea that was.

Beneath the snow, the car was entirely covered in a thick glaze. I could unlock the door with my automatic key, but the door was still frozen shut. The passenger door wouldn't budge open either. I trudged through the snow banked against the car to get to the passenger side. Both doors on that side were also glazed shut.

There was only one more way to get inside—the back door. The latch was recessed under a small ridge, so it was protected against the ice. After brushing the snow away from

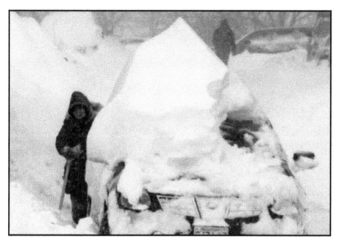

Digging out my car to go home.

the latch, I thought I was in luck. I felt my heart jump when I heard it click, but the door stayed frozen shut. I tugged on it. No movement. I got closer and gave it a heave with all the muscle I could muster. The ice cracked away from the sides, and the door opened with a creak.

Once inside, I hauled out my shovel and scraper. If I could get the car started, I thought, then the heat will help melt the door locks and defrost the ice on the windows. I lumbered over the back and fell onto the back seat. My coat was so thick I had difficulty moving.

159

This moment reminded me of when I was a child and my mother would dress me up in a one-piece quilted playsuit to go out and enjoy the snow. My gloves were pinned on the end of a string that went through the back of the snowsuit and down both sleeves. When I fell in the snow, I was so heavily dressed that I struggled to get up. I couldn't bend my knees or my arms in the quilted playsuit.

Once I was able to sit up in the backseat of the car, I waited a few minutes, wondering what to do next. Do I go head first or feet first into the driver's seat? I decided that head-first wouldn't work. I'd end up on my head and would never be able to get out of that position, so I slugged my booted foot between the front seats and balanced both hands against the backs of the front seats.

After an intimate moment with the gearshift, I was able to twist my legs over to the driver's seat. The engine groaned and protested my trying to start it.

"What if the damn thing doesn't start?" I thought. I held my breath as I gave the key another twist. It gave me a reluctant cough and then caught hold.

Once the heat was turned up and both defrosters were working, I put my hands over the vents to bring life back into them. The heating pads in my gloves helped a little but didn't send heat down into my fingers, where I needed it the most.

I was exhausted. My head fell back and my eyes closed. I stretched out my legs. God, that felt good! Maybe if I just took a short nap, I would feel better prepared to fight the elements on the road.

But in a few moments, I didn't feel better. I felt worse. My head began to swirl, and I struggled to get enough air into my lungs. It wasn't because I was tired. This was different. Something was terribly wrong. Then I knew. Carbon monoxide! The tailpipe must be blocked!

I shut off the engine and tried to open the window, but it was frozen shut. I struggled to get the door open but it wouldn't budge. I leaned back and jammed my foot against the door. Nothing. My head pounded, and my eyes stopped focusing. The door began to look blurry.

"This can't be happening," I thought. I felt panic rise up to my throat. I could feel my heart pounding against my chest and a fist tightening around my heart. With what little energy I could muster, I gave both feet a heave against the door. It creaked open an inch. I gave it another shove, and it opened, pouring a torrent of snow over me and the seat. Fresh air! I gulped in some deep breaths and staggered outside.

As I leaned against the door, my eyes and head cleared. Supporting myself against the car, I slowly made my way behind the car and bent down to look down into the tailpipe. A block of ice the size of a Coke bottle was frozen and jammed in the pipe. I now knew I couldn't drive this car home. I would have to find someone who could take me home or I would be sleeping on that miserable army cot, possibly in the cold, if the school's cranky generator quit again. I cleared away some of the snow off the car so I could find it again when I returned to claim it, whenever that would be, and stumbled back to the shelter.

Scott was just inside the door directing a couple of AmeriCorps boys to help load up the DART cages into a van. Seeing me standing inside the door, he waved. I gave a weak wave back. He walked over to me.

"You all right? Pardon me, I don't mean to be crude, but you look like hell."

I told him about my experience with the car. "Can you find me someone who can take me home? I'm tired, I haven't slept in..." I checked my watch. "...29 hours, and I'm hungry."

"Go sit down at the desk. I'll get you a cup of coffee and donuts. The EMTs brought them on their last trip to the other shelter. I know a guy who has a big old truck who can drive you home."

Scott returned with a cup of coffee and two glazed donuts. "It's black. I hope you don't mind. There's no more sugar or milk."

"I think I'm in love with you, Scott. Would your wife mind?"

"She might if I had one."

I cupped my hands around the Styrofoam cup and felt the warmth seep into my cold fingers and hands. My purple fingertips gradually pinked up. I didn't want to drink the black stuff; I just wanted to feel its warmth on my hands.

Once they warmed up, I crisscrossed my arms on the desk and rested my head on them. I willed my eyes to stay open but they had a mind of their own and closed. It felt so good to relax like that. I don't know how long I was asleep, but I woke up with a start when I felt a hand on my shoulder shaking me.

"Hey, no sleeping on the job," joked Scott.

I jumped up. "The patients! Are they all right?"

"Wake up, Terri. They have all been transferred out." He pointed to a tall, broad-shouldered man standing next to him. "This is Brad. He has a beast of a truck and said he will take you home. He doesn't mind driving you because he doesn't live far from your house."

I picked up my boat bag. "Oh bless you, Brad."

"I'll need to shovel out my truck and clean it off. Meet you at the front door in fifteen minutes." He walked out the doors and was swallowed up by the whiteness.

Chapter 17
"I CAN DO THIS, I THINK."

2:00pm

It was about twenty minutes before Brad's truck appeared. I felt like a damsel in distress who was being swooped up and carried away from danger by a knight in a shining black truck instead of on a majestic Friesian horse.

Brad had a ruddy complexion, whiskey-brown eyes, a tangle of thick brown hair that brushed against the fur on his collar, bushy eyebrows, and a thick mustache that fanned open when he smiled. I could smell the residue of smoke on his clothes. His tobacco-stained fingers turned up the windshield defroster. He lit a cigarette and tossed the glowing match into a half-full ashtray. "Hope you don't mind the smoke."

"No. My mother smoked to the day she breathed her last. I'm used to it."

He looked over at me as I grasped the sides of the open door to lift my foot inside, but the cab was too high for me to easily step up into it. As I struggled to pull myself up, I suddenly felt strong, confident hands grab hold of my jacket and yank me onto the seat.

"That was well done!" I joked.

He spoke with the cigarette bobbling up and down from the side of his mouth. "My wife has the same problem. Belt up."

Once I was seated I felt the blessed heat melting the snow off my boots. Brad turned his radio on.

After felling hundreds of trees, knocking out power to thousands of homes and ripping apart coastal dunes, the blizzard left more than forty percent of Cape households without power. Safety officials warned that it could be days before the lights were restored for everyone. More than 189,000 NStar customers throughout the Cape and Islands are left without power.

The cold drove even the hardiest Cape Codders into local shelters. It was reported that the Shelton shelter had to be closed when their generators malfunctioned after their power went out. People who sheltered there were transferred to one of the other three shelters.

He kept his eyes locked on the road in front of him as he spoke. "Looks like we're in for a long haul with this one," said Brad. "My father is a tough old bird. Was born here and never left the Cape. Didn't want to ever go over the bridge. His father had a strawberry farm just up the road where you live. I spoke to him about coming to the shelter with me, but he was skeptical. Do you know what he said?"

"He's been through storms before and came out just fine?"

"Close," he said, "And I quote, 'It ain't ever as bad as the weather guys always say it's gonna to be. I've been through this more times than a frog hops on the hot tarmac. Everyone gets all worked up, and then it just fizzles out. He has a fireplace and enough wood to keep him warm for the entire winter. He believes it's important to be able to make it on your own."

I removed my gloves and put my hands close to the hot air blowing out the vents. "Tough guy. Typical old Cape Codder. Can't blame him for that."

"He's tough, all right, but guess what he said after a few hours into this storm." Brad didn't wait for me to respond. He said, "This one's gonna be a doozy.'"

The snow swirled in front of the truck, making it look like we were being sucked through a perpetual swirling vortex. He kept talking. "Looks like they've plowed the main roads. It's the side roads I'm worried about. Is your road a town road?"

"It never got picked up by the town because it is still zoned as farm land. There are only twelve houses on it. It was once part of an old turkey farm, so I don't know why they called it Bacon Farm Road. When I first moved there, my neighbor had a goat, a pigmy pig, and a rooster. Every morning, as the first sliver of light peeked over the horizon, that rooster started crowing. I was working the evening shift at the time. I got home at 12:30

at night. I'd play with the dogs, get something to eat, and then I'd read to make my eyes tired so I could sleep. I'd go to bed around 1:30 and be asleep for about three to four hours when that old rooster started crowing. I'd try to sleep with a pillow over my head. I blessed the day it headed to the great chicken coop in the sky."

"So who plows your road?"

"My neighbor is the fire chief, so someone from the fire department comes around with a plow. There are only 150 steps from the beginning of the road to my house."

"How do you know that?"

"I've counted them when I go out for a walk."

The truck skidded a bit as he turned the corner off route 28, the road that was a mile from the turnoff to my house. When he came to my road, he stopped. "Your road hasn't been plowed. The drifts are well over my bumper. I'm sorry, but I can't chance getting stuck. I'm going to have to leave you off here to walk the short distance home."

"No problem, Brad. I appreciate your help in getting me this far." I opened the door and dropped down into a three-foot-high bank of snow. I slung the bag over my shoulder and waved him off.

Then I turned to face my road. It was covered in snowdrifts so high that there was no way to distinguish the road from the surrounding terrain. The scene was straight out of a *National Geographic* feature on the frozen landscape of northern Alaska. The snow was up to my thighs. The wind felt like icy fingers scraping the snow across the softness of my cheeks."

I pulled my scarf over my cheeks and tucked the sides into my jacket. "One hundred and fifty steps," I said to myself, and took a deep breath. I let it out slowly between pursed lips.

"I can do this," I said quietly to the universe.

Chapter 18
THE LONG ROAD HOME

3:00pm

I turned to face the landscape in front of me. It seemed like I was staring into another world. The wind raced along the surface of the snow, stinging any area of my skin that was exposed. I felt the icy snow seeping into my boots and starting to melt. I had to start moving and get some warmth into my feet before my wet socks started to freeze.

By then, I hadn't slept in 31 hours. Every muscle in my body ached, and I could barely focus on the task ahead. Could I really do this? With luck and a prayer for help, I faced the road and started to move.

I tried to pick up my right leg for my first giant step, but it wouldn't move. I gave it another heave. It slipped out from the tight grip of the snow. One step. Great! Only 149 more to go. I tugged my left leg up and extended it as far up as I could to get above the snow level. Two steps. I looked ahead to see the

171

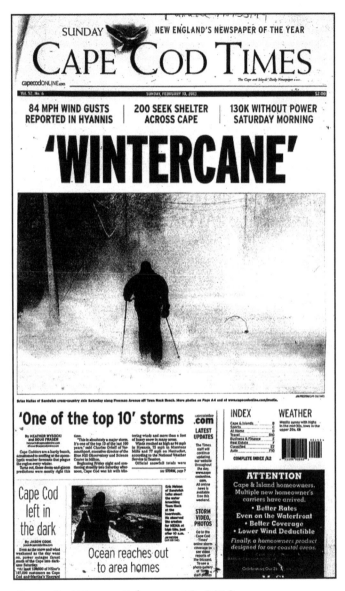

Cape Cod Times, February 10, 2013

bend in the road. I guessed it would be about half way, so seventy-five steps from where I stood. Another lift of my right leg and then my left. Each leg sank deep into the piled-up snow ahead of me and dared me to move it again.

My boat bag slapped against my side with every step. It felt heavier than when I first brought it into the shelter. How could that be? All the food that was in it was gone. Twenty steps. I pulled the bag off my shoulder and tossed it ahead of me on top on the snow. I struggled with another step, picked up the bag and repeated the move with every step.

There were three houses lined up on my right. What if I made it to one of those houses and asked to be let in to warm up? Maybe take a short nap. The first house was about ten steps back from where I stood. I stared at the windows, looking for movement inside. Nothing. The lights were off, but then again, maybe the power was out. What if I wasted ten steps to the house and no one was there? I would have wasted twenty steps only to be back where I am now. With no obvious signs of life in the house, I decided against taking the chance.

One hundred and ten more steps. The wind whipped my hood off. Snow fell around my head and neck and melted down my back. When I flipped it back up, more snow fell over my face. I shivered and wrapped my woolen scarf a little tighter around my neck and over my cheeks. I tried to wriggle my toes but couldn't feel them. The Reynaud's in my feet had been triggered by the cold, wet socks. My fingers were also numb. The little heat packs were helping but didn't radiate the heat down into my fingers, where I needed it the most.

Only fifteen more steps to go before I reached the half way point. My legs and arms were numb. What if I don't make it? I pondered. What did it feel like to freeze to death? I had heard it really wasn't so bad. I heard that people just fall asleep and never wake up.

I remembered from my training as an emergency room nurse that if a person's body temperature drops from the normal 98.6F degrees to about 95F, the body begins to shut down. My body shivered with the cold.

"This feels awful, but it's a good sign," I thought. "It means my body is trying to compensate for the cold." But not feeling my hands and feet was not a good sign. It might mean they were in danger of frostbite.

Seventy-five more steps. I was almost halfway there. I came to the curve in the road. I could barely catch my breath. Suddenly, my feet slipped out backwards from under me, and my upper body fell flat out onto the snow.

The road was covered with a layer of ice under the snow. I remembered how I was always careful when driving on this curve in bad weather because for some reason, it was almost always slippery with ice in the winter, rain in the summer, and wet leaves in the fall.

I tried to push myself up, but my hands sank deeper into the snow, and my feet kept slipping out from under me on the ice below. It felt like being imprisoned in quicksand. Struggling only made me sink deeper into the snow. I had nothing solid to balance myself against or to or to help me stand.

I stopped struggling. It felt so good to just lie there. Maybe I could just take a short nap and then try again once I regained my strength. Then I remembered the instructor in my emergency room certification class saying,

"In hypothermia, heart and breathing rates slow down accompanied with confusion and sleepiness. As your body temperature drops, your heart, brain, and internal organs cannot function."

I couldn't stay here. Somehow, I had to get up and keep taking steps, but I couldn't move.

My mind went back to an incident one that happened in October. At around 12:30am, when I left the hospital after working an evening shift. I am not always compliant about putting on my seat belt, and that night as no different. My excuse was that at this time of night and during the off-season on the Cape, the road was usually deserted.

I turned on the audio of a book I was listening to. I was often able to finish a book every two weeks by doing this. When I started my car, an intense feeling came over me. I felt a strong urge to put my seat belt on, shut off the audio, and be hyper-vigilant while driving. About what?

I tried to shrug it off. This made no sense, but the feeling was so overwhelming that I couldn't ignore it. So I did what my intuition was telling me to do and began the 45-minute drive home from Hyannis to Falmouth. I was careful to stay within the speed limit. I gripped the wheel with both hands. Like a soldier searching for a hidden enemy, I scrutinized everything around me as I drove down the road to Falmouth.

I passed the shopping malls and saw nothing unusual. The road was void of traffic and lit by a full moon that shone like a pearl.

"Remember me," my mother used to say. "Remember me when you see the full moon. That will be me smiling down on you." My mother's name was Pearl.

A half-hour later I circled the Mashpee rotary, passed two exits, and took the road that led me into Falmouth. I was only ten minutes away from home. My shoulders ached from the tension.

"This makes no sense," I reasoned. "What am I expecting?" I chided myself for being foolish enough to believe, with no obvious proof, that some unknown danger was lurking out there. Dread? Fear? Of what? I was working myself up for nothing.

I relaxed my shoulders and hands and slumped a bit back into my seat.

A few miles past the Mashpee rotary, I came to a darkened area where the street was lined with trees but nothing else — no buildings or streetlights. Then I noticed two lights eerily floating in the darkness in the road ahead of me at the level of my car. They danced silently, autonomously, detached from anything. I was mesmerized watching them.

Suddenly, I realized what I was seeing! Instantly, I twisted the steering wheel to the right and landed on a grassy shoulder just as a car going in the wrong direction in my lane sped past me. I shook with fear. I had been a split second away from being hit head on.

My first reaction was anger. I wanted to turn around and follow this car that almost took my life, then call the police. But I couldn't do it. Instead, I just called the police and told about the incident of the car driving in the wrong direction.

I sat there trying to understand what had just happened. Had I not been warned, I probably would have been listening to my audio book and not been prepared for the danger waiting for me. It was an existential moment. I was keenly aware that I would remember this for the rest of my life.

Who or what warned me? And why? Was my life meant to be saved for some other purpose? What purpose would that be? I put my head against the steering wheel and offered a prayer of gratitude to God, my mother, or whoever was responsible, for saving my life. It just wasn't my time.

As I lay trapped in the snow, I offered another prayer for help. If there was a purpose then for my life to continue, wasn't there still a purpose? I don't think we know the strength inside us until everything around us gets stripped away and some primitive internal force fights for self preservation.

I picked up my head and looked all around me. There was a branch near me that had fallen from one of the overhead trees. I reached for it, but it was just beyond my grasp. I took my boat bag and hanging onto one of the handles, I tossed it to the branch. It landed on top of the branch, making it possible for me to pull it to me. I snapped off the little side twigs, stuck it in the snow, and tested my weight on it. It held. Leaning on it, I was able to hoist myself up. It worked! I could use it as a walking stick. Seventy-five more steps to home.

I could hear my instructor's voice once again. "You can get frostbite on your nose, chin, and ears as well as your fingers and toes. Try to keep them covered, but if you notice that you're having numbness or tingling or burning, you need to seek help immediately."

Get help? Who should I call for help? No one can drive down this road, let alone walk. I pulled out my phone. I was reluctant to take my glove off to tap in the security passcode, but I had no choice. I knew I couldn't make the remaining seventy-five steps.

I was weak. Tired. Numb. Every muscle in my body screamed for me to stop. My fingers were so numb I never felt the glass screen as I tapped in the numbers. But the phone wouldn't open up. I tapped them in again. Nothing.

The battery was dead. Not being able to use my phone in the shelter, I had forgotten to keep it charged. Whatever juice was left in the battery was sucked out by the cold. I shoved it back into my coat pocket. I had no choice now. I had to keep moving.

I was around the curve and could see the lights glowing in my house. I knew Elaine was waiting for me, not knowing I was only 60 steps away and struggling to reach her. I felt like a robot. I couldn't concentrate or feel my body. Everything was numb and stiff with the cold. As I got closer to home, the height of the snow dropped to the level of my knees making it easier to take the next steps.

Only 20 more steps to go. I reached the bottom of my driveway, which was on a steep incline. These would be the hardest 20 steps I'd ever taken. I started up the hill and slid back. I tried again, but I couldn't gain any traction.

"I think I can. I think I can." The memory of these words tumbled through my mind. When I was a child, my mother bought me a 45rpm record of the *Little Engine That Could.* She snapped a red adapter in the middle of the record so it would fit the spool on the turntable. It was about a train whose mission was to bring a load of toys to children on the other side of the mountain, but suddenly the engine

181

quit and it couldn't pull the load up the mountain. The children would not get their toys.

Then another, much older engine came alongside of the first train. When it was asked to take over for the first engine, it said, "I'm tired. I cannot."

A much smaller engine came by and said it was too small to pull such a big load, but when it thought of the children not getting their toys, it said it would try. It puffed and strained up the mountain all the while saying, "I think I can. I think I can."

Finally, it made it over the top of the mountain, and sliding down on the other side, it cried, "I thought I could! I thought I could!" I loved that record and played it over and over again.

"I know I can," I said out loud to the universe.

I dropped my bag, dug my walking stick into the snow, and pulled myself up the hill. Ten more steps. I came to Elaine's car in the driveway and hung on to the car handle for support.

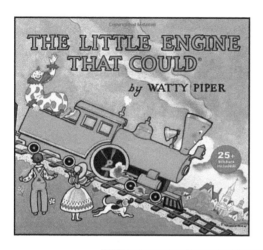

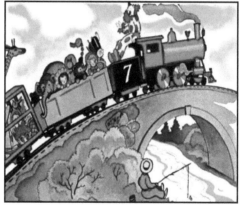

Original illustrations from the original edition of
The Little Engine that Could.

Five more steps brought me to my deck. I tripped on the step up, fell to my knees, and crawled the final five steps to the glass sliders. I rapped on the glass with my branch. Looking up, I saw two almond-shaped, yellow eyes peering out at me from the other side of the door.

Jackson rubbed against the glass and mouthed a silent hello to me. Then Elaine came to the door, saw me lying on the deck, opened the slider, and screamed. "Oh, my God, Terri! Are you all right? I called the shelter, and they said you left hours ago! What are you doing on the ground? Are you hurt?"

"C...can't talk."

My whole body shook.

"S..so c...c...cold."

I managed to crawl in and get myself up into a sitting position.

"P...p...please. Have t...to warm up."

She reached down and pulled me up. I fell into her arms. I was home.

Chapter 19
WHO IS SHE?

One week later

The Red Cross staff gathered once a month to catch up on the news, share our experiences, and learn about any updates. This was the first meeting since the storm. The air was charged with excitement. Before the meeting was called to order, people gathered around a table positioned along one side of the room and covered with an array of pizza boxes and cans of Pepsi. I could hear snippets of conversations as people shared their shelter experiences during the storm.

"Yeah, I stayed for two days until they..."

"They opened ours up when the Shelton patrons..."

"We got lasagna. You only got bagels?"

"DART got four dogs, three cats, and a ferret at our shelter."

I stood next to Max, who had been a faithful Red Cross staffer for many years. He was in his sixties and had a head of thick, snow-white hair and a mustache that danced on his upper lip when he talked. He supervised many of the training classes.

When I had first joined the Red Cross six years before, we had a run-in that almost ended my willingness to be a part of this organization.. When I missed one of his classes, he threatened to drop me.

"You took the place of someone else that I had to turn away because of space. If you aren't going to be responsible, the Red Cross doesn't need you."

I felt my face flare. "I had to put my dog, Tucker, to sleep today. He had liver cancer. Do you think I wanted to have to do that? Should I have left him alone, bleeding rectally on the rug, and let him suffer and die while I attended your class? What kind of person are you that you would think your class was more important than having to put my dog down? Believe me, Max, I would have much preferred to attend your class."

There was silence on the other end of the phone. "Well, okay. Sorry. I'll let you go through just this once."

He eased up on me after that, but the relationship was always edgy until we shared a shelter assignment. After that, we gained a mutual respect for each other and became good friends. I often turned to him when I had a question or needed an explanation of something happening with the Red Cross.

I learned that this organization is vast and complex and always under construction. I often had trouble trying to keep up with the changes. Max was a straight-from-the-shoulder kind of guy and always told me what he thought without mincing words.

"So what shelter did you work in during the storm?" I asked him.

"I worked the one in Yarmouth. I've been there before. We were the busiest shelter of the four. I was there for three days. That was a rough assignment. Longest time I've had to work a shelter. The hospital was also inundated with people for all kinds of problems — broken bones, back strain, and chest pains.

"What was unusual was that over 30 people were admitted to the ER because they were unable to maintain their oxygen levels when the power went out in their homes. They were all on oxygen concentrators.

"Weren't you at the Shelton shelter? What happened there?"

I put a slice of pepperoni pizza on my flimsy paper plate, picked up a can of Pepsi, and motioned for him to sit with me. "It was a challenge. We struggled to keep two people breathing who were on oxygen when the back-up generator kept failing. There also was woman with a feeding-tube pump that was shut off for most of the night and a woman with pica who required a CPAP machine to breathe when sleeping.

"Oh yeah, also, there was no heat and barely any food. Just bagels. I had a bitch of a shelter manager who wouldn't work with me or the MRC nurse to move these people out to a safer place. She acted like she was an army sergeant. We had to call the head of the EMS to get her to transfer people out to the shelter they opened up."

"I heard about that. Lucky you! You got to go home earlier than the rest of us."

"Yeah, well that's a story for another time." I decided not to tell him my saga of trying to get home.

He raised the corner of his pizza to his lips. "Who was your shelter manager?"

"Someone named Pat McNutter. Do you know who she is?"

Just then, the Cape Cod Red Cross chapter administrator tapped on the microphone. "Take your seats please. This meeting will now come to order. We have a lot of information to cover and we all want to go home on time."

"Later," Max whispered to me.

The administrator read from her notes. "The storm left more than 189,000 people in the cold and dark. All four of our shelters were full and stayed that way until the storm was over. Shelters are a vital component of our emergency system to keep people safe during storms like this."

"I leaned over to Max and whispered, "You'd never know it from the shelter manager I dealt with."

The administrator gave me one of those looks you got from your fourth-grade teacher when you whispered in class. She cleared her throat and continued. "Although Cape Codders see themselves as a self-reliant breed, this storm has served as a reminder of just how fragile we really are. I think one of our shortcomings is that we didn't open up enough shelters. Members of the emergency committee have taken a lot of flack in the ensuing days and weeks, but the truth is that no one realized how big this storm was going to be until we were in the middle of it."

She paused, shuffled some of her papers, then looked up and continued. "After I finish with the business of this meeting, I invite you to stand up and share your experiences or ask any questions."

She went on to discuss changes in some of the forms used to evaluate people who needed financial help. There were changes in the formatting of finding where and how many volunteers were needed and how they signed up for their assignment. (I learned early on that there were always computer changes.)

Max leaned over and whispered one of his usual cryptic remarks. "I'm a military veteran. I thought the army was the most mismanaged organization in America until I worked for the Red Cross."

I wrote back on the agenda paper to avoid getting the evil eye again from the moderator. "Maybe, but you're still here. You either love it or you're a glutton for punishment. "

He took the pen and paper from me and wrote back, "I'm here for the same reason you are."

The administrator sat down and opened up the meeting for people to share their experiences. A few used this time to thank others for their help. One man praised the AmeriCorps kids for volunteering their much-needed help. "America will be a better country when these kids grow up and become our leaders," he said. "Let's all give them a hand." He got a loud round of applause.

Someone else liked the article written by the journalist who had spoken to Jan Holloway. After everyone else was done speaking, I stood up.

"This was my fourth shelter experience of setting up the medical clinic. It was also my most disturbing and difficult assignment." There was a hush over the audience. "The feeling that we put lives at risk when the power went out and the generators didn't start up still haunts me."

I went on to tell them my experience at the Shelton shelter.

"The shelter manager would not under any circumstances move these patients to a safer place until she was forced to when Jan called Stan Lawrence, the head of the CCES. He was the one who ordered the transfers of the most critical patients first and then the shelter shutdown. I thank God for him. I hope this situation can be dealt with and resolved so that it never happens again. I know that neither Jan nor I will ever work under this manager again. She put people's lives at risk."

When I sat down, no one spoke. No one moved. One person covered up a cough. They just sat with their eyes fixed on the administrator, who cleared her throat again. "I'll discuss this with Alice Kent-Levinson, Chief Nurse of our Red Cross Chapter." She rapped her knuckles on the table. "Meeting is dismissed."

Max turned to me. "I need to talk to you. You are going to get into a heap of trouble if you mess with McNutter. They won't remove her."

"Why? Who is she?"

Suddenly the administrator appeared. "Sorry, I need to steal this handsome silver fox from you, Terri." She put her arm around Max's shoulder and steered him away from me. "Max, can we take a few minutes to discuss the next set of classes? I have some people interested in attending and Lord knows, we need all the volunteers we can get."

Max looked back at me. "Talk to you later," he said over his shoulder as he disappeared into the crowd of people who were still milling around.

Chapter 20
"JUST LET THIS GO."

Five days later

I glanced over the headlines of the *Boston Globe* just before I was about to prepare a quick lunch. Then I folded the paper in half to read some of the story.

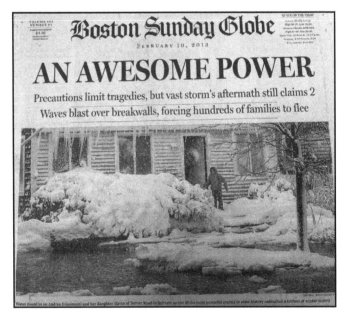

Boston Sunday Globe, February 10, 2013

POWER FAILURE

Pummeled by one of the worst winter storms in state history, much of Massachusetts spent the weekend digging out, waiting for power, and navigating a snow-shrouded landscape that proved both pristinely beautiful and savagely cruel. Two people died and two were injured with carbon-monoxide poisoning linked to the storm which dumped more than 30 inches of snow in the state. Hundreds of coastal residents were evacuated from the North Shore to Cape Cod. More than 400,000 people in Massachusetts alone awoke without power Saturday. Governor Deval Patrick lifted the statewide travel ban on...

The phone rang.

"Hey, Terri, it's Alice."

I put the newspaper aside and the phone on speaker so I could continue to make my ham salad sandwich. "Hi, Alice. I could never mistake that New York accent for anyone else but you."

"I'm calling you because the moderator asked me talk to you. She said you were very upset about your Shelton shelter experience and is very concerned that you discussed it as last week's monthly meeting."

I put the phone between my cheek and shoulder, opened up the refrigerator door, and a placed a loaf of bread and a container of ham salad on the counter.

"Is she more concerned about what happened or that I shared it at the meeting?"

"Both."

I put the phone on the counter and opened the twist tie on the loaf of multi-grained bread.

"She should be concerned about what happened at the Shelton shelter. I sure am. You should be too. As for sharing it at the meeting, which the moderator requested by the way, I think it was very appropriate for everyone to know what happened. Why not?"

"She thought you should have come to her first before you opened it up to all of the staff."

"Well, here's the deal. It took me a few days to recover from the trip home. One of the EMTs dropped me off at the start of my street because it was unplowed. I had to walk 150 steps in thigh-high snow to get to my house in the blizzard, while bucking hurricane winds. I think the only reason why I didn't get frost-bite was because when I finally got home,

Elaine immediately put me in a tub of luke-warm water to defrost my hands and feet. It took me two days to recover from that. I was lucky I didn't get pneumonia."

"I'm sorry that happened. You could have stayed in the shelter."

"You mean the one that had no heat, food or anyone else but the maintenance man?"

"You still could have called the moderator when you felt better or you could have waited until after the meeting to discuss this with her."

"When Governor Patrick lifted the travel ban, Elaine drove me back to the high school to get my car. It was completely buried. We both worked half of the day to dig it out. Just to add more to the fun, once the car was dug out, I had to chip out a block of ice from my tailpipe the size of a soda can. Oh, and did I mention that I almost died from carbon monoxide poisoning when I started the car, not knowing the tailpipe was blocked?

"There was no time to call the moderator, and besides, I was still trying to decide what to do about the whole experience."

I put two slices of bread in the toaster.

"Could you have waited until after the meeting?"

"After the meeting she cornered Max, and I never saw either of them again. Look, she needed to know that that shelter manager put people's lives at risk. McNutter was impossible to deal with and made no attempt to help our patients, all the while dumping the total responsibility for them on Jan and myself. If someone had died, who would have been responsible for it?"

"You would. You were the nurse in charge of the clinic."

I threw the knife in the sink.

"I would? I would be responsible, when I had no power to do what was needed to help these people? Patients could have died or suffered serious medical complications, and both Jan and I could have lost our nursing licenses and it's all my fault?

"I asked to have them evacuated to the hospital. I can't produce oxygen out of thin air or rub two sticks together for heat. McNutter refused everything I asked for. She had all of the control."

"Of course. She was in charge of the shelter."

"Alice, can you hear yourself? You are saying that while Jan and I were responsible for the patients under our care, we had no say as to how to keep them safe, but we were still medically and legally responsible for them if they got into trouble."

"You could have called an ambulance and had them transferred to the hospital."

The toast popped up. I picked up the tossed knife out of the sink and popped open the plastic lid on the container of ham salad.

"No, we couldn't! The ambulance drivers and EMTs were answered to McNutter. They wouldn't do anything without her permission. Someone had to have the authority to call in a larger plow so they could get out of the driveway. That would be McNutter's responsibility."

"But a larger plow was sent in and cleared the way for the ambulance to get to the hospital. So what was the problem?"

I piled ham salad onto the toast.

"She should have called Stan Lawrence, the head of the Cape's Coalition of Emergency Services for help, but she didn't. Jan had to do it. That's how we got the larger plow. Do you know why she didn't call him and ask for help — aside from her giant ego getting in her way?"

"No, why?"

"Because she didn't know who he was! That's why. Jan had to overrule her and intervene. The truth is that McNutter refused to work with us to keep these people safe. She should have sent the 90-year-old woman, who couldn't sleep on the army cot and had infected lower legs, to the hospital. That was an inappropriate admission. She should have called for back-up oxygen tanks. And when she couldn't get the damn back-up generator to work, we had no heat. She should have made plans to evacuate everyone."

"When you called me, I spoke to her, and she said she was sure the generator would come back on."

"Sure, but when and for how long? It went on and then went off again. And while we were waiting, I watched two COPDers oxygen saturation drop down below 90% and everyone huddling under blankets to keep warm."

I cut the sandwich in half.

"If that wasn't problem enough, she deliberately evacuated the less urgent patients first and the most urgent patients last. And while we were evacuating people, she actually admitted a woman who was in worse shape than anyone we already had there. She should have just put her on the ambulance to the hospital or the shelter where everyone was being transferred to.

"Look, Alice. I have worked for you many times over the years and admire all that you do. You are an outstanding member of the Red Cross, and you have been doing it for years. In addition to your working with the local chapter, you have also been deployed numerous times to various disasters in other states. They can't give you a raise because you have been working as a volunteer. They should be giving you the Henry Dunant Medal—did I get the name right? Wasn't he the founder of the Red Cross movement?"

"I believe so."

"You should have gotten it in honor for all that you do for them. Maybe you didn't understand the totality of this situation at the Shelton shelter. God only knows, you had your hands full those three days."

"I'm sorry this happened, Terri. There will be a monthly meeting of the Cape's Coalition of Emergency Services in a week to review any problems. It will be brought up there. But you do know that the Red Cross provides liability coverage to their nurses and other emergency staff."

"And how does that work?"

"Give me a minute and I'll have the wording."

I heard papers being shuffled in the background.

"Here it is." She began to read. "Laws shielding volunteers from liability have been enacted on both the federal and state level."

"It goes on to say, 'This statute provides immunity so long as the volunteer was acting within the scope of his or her responsibilities, and the volunteer was licensed or certified in the state where the harm occurred, if licensure or certification was required.'"

I brought the sandwich over to the table and set a cup of water into the microwave to heat for tea.

"That's nice, but little relief if a patient is lost on my watch. I want to be at the CCES meeting. I want to explain to them what happened and ask how we can prevent it from happening again."

Alice's voice faltered. "You...you can't be there. You aren't on the committee."

"Invite me as a guest."

"I can't do that. These monthly meetings are attended only by specific people who are in charge of various agencies that provide emergency services on the Cape. You know, Terri, you should just let this drop. You gave your concerns at the monthly Red Cross meeting. That should be enough."

"No, Alice, it's not. McNutter has to be confronted with what she did, and the CCSC needs to be sure she is never put in charge of another shelter."

"I'll bring up your issues about her, but I don't think they will withdraw her from working the shelters."

"Why? For God's sake, who is she? Jesus Christ, Superstar? No one in the shelter knew who she was. She had no emergency, disaster, shelter, or medical experience, but there she was, totally inadequate but still running the show as if she were an army platoon sergeant in charge of regimental Company B."

The whirr of the microwave stopped, and it beeped three times, announcing that its job was done. When I took the cup out and turned around, my cat had jumped up on the counter and was eating the ham salad out of the sandwich.

I waved him away. "Scoot, Jackson. I know it's time for your lunch. I'll get it for you in a minute." With that, he turned and kicked off with his back feet, knocking the dish and sandwich to the tile floor. The ham salad splattered, and the dish shattered into white shards over the floor.

"Look, you're busy," said Alice. "Go have your lunch and leave the rest to me. I do want to remind you again that the Red Cross does carry liability insurance for its staff and volunteers. If I can bring you to the meeting, I'll give you a call."

"No rush. My cat just knocked my sandwich on the floor. I need to tell you one last thing before we hang up. I will never work under McNutter again. Jan said she wouldn't either. Not only that, but she won't send any of her MRC nurses to work under her. And when you send one of your other nurses,

204

you'll have the same problem again. How far does it have to go before we remove her? Does someone have to die first? Oh, that's right. I forgot. It will be the nurse's fault," I said, sarcasm dripping from my voice.

"Terri, I appreciate everything you've done for the Red Cross over the years. You have agreed to do anything I've asked you to do without complaint. I enjoy working with you. You have been more than just a member of this organization. I also consider you a friend, so I feel badly that you are so upset over this. I'll do my best. I probably shouldn't tell you this, but because of our friendship, I will. They won't remove her, and it's best for all of us, especially the Red Cross, if you just let this go."

With that, the phone went dead.

Chapter 21
WHO YOU ARE DEALING WITH

One month later

It was time for our monthly meeting with the Red Cross staff. Alice never called me back about the region-wide emergency services meeting. I didn't have to guess why she didn't.

There was no pizza for this Red Cross meeting but someone did bring in a few boxes of Dunkin' Donuts doughnuts and containers of Cup 'O Joe. I looked for a decaf coffee, but there was none, so I poured a cup of the high-test coffee, knowing I would have to double up on my Tums when I got home. As I was about to pick up a Boston cream doughnut, a hairy hand crossed mine.

"You can't have that one," said a male voice behind me. "It's my favorite doughnut and this is the last one."

I turned around to see Max's open smile.

"Just kidding. I couldn't eat it if I wanted to. I'm a diabetic." He wrapped it up in a napkin. As he handed it to me, it fell out of the napkin onto the floor. When I reached down to pick it up, I noticed he was wearing open-toed sandals.

"Max, why aren't you wearing shoes. It's 39 degrees outside."

He picked his foot up and looked like he was inspecting it for the first time. "My legs and feet are swollen. My shoes were too tight, and the sandals are the only footwear I could be comfortable in. You're the nurse. What do you think this is?"

"I don't know you well enough to guess. It could be any of a dozen things, like congestive heart failure, peripheral vascular disease, or kidney failure. None of it is good. Are you being followed by a doctor for your diabetes?"

"Oh, sure, he has been following my blood sugar and kidney tests. He is concerned about the kidney tests. Says if they don't improve I may have to go on dialysis."

Max waited while I threw the dropped doughnut away and grabbed another one; then we walked over to find a place where we could sit together. I found two folding chairs in the last row, opened them up, and offered one to Max. "I'm sorry to hear that dialysis might be a possibility. I hope it doesn't come to that, but if it does, let me know if there's anything I can do for you."

He pulled another folding chair up in front of him, put his feet up on it, and took a sip of his coffee. "To change the subject," he said. "How did you make out at the Regional Emergency Meeting last month?"

"I didn't. I'm not invited to attend that meeting. Only important people go, and I'm not that important."

"I'm not surprised. After every disaster, about 15 to 18 people, representing various agencies, like the town health agents, head of the EMS, police chief, fire chief, and head of the Red Cross, Salvation Army officers, and more, give what they call an 'After Action Report.'

"Alice probably doesn't go to those meetings. The only way she can handle your shelter manager problem is if she gives the information to the Red Cross representative, and they report it. She may have tried to explain what happened but I get the feeling she would rather have had a root canal during her colonoscopy, both without anesthesia, than to discuss the Shelton shelter manager problem at that meeting. The press goes to these monthly meetings, so the people there suppress any negative comments."

Max took another sip of his coffee and then held it in his lap.

"I'm not surprised. She knows they won't do anything about McNutter, and she doesn't want to be caught up in the drama."

I took a bite out of my doughnut. "Cut the mystery, Max. Tell me..."

"Let's all take our seats, please. We have a lot to discuss tonight," said the administrator as she rapped her knuckle on the microphone, which squealed in protest.

The meeting proceeded with the usual issues: a new admissions form had been placed on the computer. People were having problems trying to log onto the Red Cross site (I was one of them). She directed the discussion to a volunteer who was called in to help the two families displaced by an apartment fire. The woman described how she placed them in a local hotel, gave them credit cards for food, medications, and in the case of one family, supplies for a baby and referred them to social services to follow up on their needs.

Another man stood up to say that his Red Cross ERV (Emergency Rescue Vehicle) ran out of food during the apartment fire and needed to be resupplied. There was a discussion that since the Cape Red Cross chapter no longer stood alone but was now bundled in with the entire southeastern district of Massachusetts, the central office had decided that the Cape, with it relatively low population, didn't need three ERVs.

"They took one of our ERVs to be used off-Cape," said a man who was plainly upset. "We were told that if we joined in with the southeastern district, they would provide us with more services and equipment, not less. It will now take us twice as long to get from Hyannis to Falmouth or Dennis or Harwich to P'town. It isn't about the population. It's about the geography of the Cape and the congestion on the roads during the tourist season, but you can't get an off-Caper to understand this."

"We've discussed this with the district coordinator more than once," said the administrator. "But unfortunately we could not persuade him to leave our three ERVs on the

Cape," There was a mumble of dissatisfaction among the crowd.

Finally, the meeting was over.

Max took the last gulp of coffee and crushed the cup in his hand. "Can I talk to you about what to expect if the decision is made to put me on dialysis? I don't know anything about how it all works."

"Sure. Call me tonight if you are up to it."

As soon as I walked in the door at home, the phone rang. It was Max. He wanted to know everything there was to know about having dialysis. I asked him to give me a minute to take my coat off and get settled.

I gave Elaine a hug and whispered that I needed to take this call. Elaine motioned that supper was being kept warm in the oven. Picking the phone back up, I explained to him that I had been in charge of a cardiac/renal unit where they treated people who required dialysis. "So I had some good experience with the process," I said.

I tried to make the information as simple as possible to understand. "To undergo dialysis, you would first need to have a surgical procedure called an A-V fistula in your lower arm. This provides a place for the dialysis machine to connect with your vascular system. Placing it is considered minor surgery..."

"Minor if it's not their arm," Max broke in.

"Look, Max. Why don't you take this one step at a time? You may not need this. There is also another method called peritoneal dialysis, that can be done at home through the abdomen. You don't know yet if you'll need either of them. Hopefully you won't. Let me know what your renal doctor says."

Elaine put out the dinner plates and pointed to her watch, suggesting that it was time to get off the phone and eat the supper she had prepared. I mouthed, "Wait just a few minutes," and turned back to the phone.

The silence on the other end was long enough for me to think either the call had been dropped or he had hung up. I wondered if all of this was too overwhelming for him to absorb. Then his voice came back on.

"I owe you a favor for this, and, if I have to go one dialysis, I'll be calling on you in the future to explain more about this to me. As for the other problem, with the Shelton shelter, I think you have a right to know. I may get in trouble for telling you this, but I will tell you anyways. You didn't hear this from me, okay?"

I sat at the table that was already set for supper. "Okay. I agree. So tell me, what's up?"

"The shelter manager you were having problems with..." His voice dropped off and then came back again. "...you need to know who you are dealing with."

My throat tightened. "Who might that be?"

"She's the sister of Shelton's fire chief. Her brother was able to get her the job because he attends all of the monthly emergency meetings. Of all of the volunteers and staff, the shelter manager is the only one who gets paid."

"That's not a good reason to allow her to do this, and God only knows what other damage she could do in the future because of her ignorance and overinflated ego."

Elaine started to pour iced tea into glasses and to dole out a steaming portion of poached salmon, topped with a generous scoop of buttered bread crumbs.

"Thank you for this, Max, but I have to go..."

"That's not all," he interrupted. "She's also married to the district court judge. If the Red Cross creates a problem with her, not only will they be subject to legal suits but because of her husband, no lawyer will touch the case."

"So she felt confident enough to warn us not to cross the line with her because she knew no one could hold her responsible for her decisions."

Elaine filled the rest of the plate with jasmine rice and steamed broccoli, smothered in cheese sauce. Just then Jackson jumped up on my lap and put his nose to the salmon on my plate. I picked him off my lap and put him on the floor. "No, you can't do that."

"Do what?" asked Max. "I'm not going to do anything, and neither are you."

"No, not you. My cat, who just had his nose in my dinner plate."

"One more thing, and then you can go eat your supper. Here's the final kicker. Her son works for the Chamber of Commerce. He directs businesses to donate financial gifts and grants to many of the agencies the Emergency

Services deal with. If we pull her from this position, we will also lose a considerable number of much-needed donations."

It was my turn to be speechless. "I...don't know what to say ... except it's worse than I imagined. So that's why I'm getting so much resistance to the idea that we should remove her, or even discuss the problem?"

"Promise you won't tell anyone I told you this, and for everyone's sake, including your own, let it go."

I made the promise, then hung up and sat there stunned. Elaine saw the look on my face. She came over and put her hand on my shoulder. "You look awful. Can I get you something?"

"No, just give me a minute to process what I just heard."

"Do you want me to reheat your supper?"

I took a sip of the iced tea. It helped relieve the lump in my throat.

"Just give me a few minutes. Then I'll explain everything at supper." I put my cell phone down, but it slid off the table and onto the floor. Jackson, who was still sitting by my chair, went over and flopped on top of it. I fished it out from under him and patted his soft gray fur. He turned his head up for me to scratch under his chin. "I'll save you some salmon after the meal," I promised him.

Elaine sat down across from me. "Is it all right for me to ask what is upsetting you so much, or would you rather we discussed it after supper?"

"For now, let's just enjoy this beautiful meal you cooked."

The next few minutes of silence were broken by Jackson, who protested that he wasn't getting his share of the salmon fast enough. Elaine picked up the 17-pound cat and put him on his favorite rug by the door. "If you don't stop begging for food from the table, we'll have to enroll you in Jenny Craig."

I reached down and gave him a pinch of catnip to take him mind off of the salmon.

She pointed at me. "And if you don't stop drugging him with catnip, we'll also have to enroll him in a Suboxone clinic."

She sat down, picked up a hot, crispy roll, and took a bite. Melted butter dripped down the side of her hand. She hesitated, trying to decide whether to lick it off or use a napkin.

Knowing she was tidy about everything, I bet the napkin would be her choice; I was right. After she cleaned her hand up, I put my hand on hers to get her attention. "Have you ever heard the saying, 'You can't control the wind, but you can adjust the sails?' "

"No. What does that mean?"

"It's the Cape Cod way of saying when you can't control what's happening, challenge yourself to control the way you respond to what's happening. That's where the power and control is."

Chapter 22
ONE MORE THING

The next day

After making a quick breakfast on our new waffle iron, Elaine left for her job working in the Activities Department of an assistive living facility. I cleaned up, then I phoned Alice.

"Hey, Alice. It's Terri. Is this a good time to talk to you?"

"I have to leave for the Red Cross center in about a half-hour so sure. What's up?"

"Alice..." I hesitated searching for the right words but decided to just put it on the line. "Here's the thing. I now know who Pat McNutter is and why no one wants to deal with her atrocious behavior at the shelter and why she won't be removed."

Silence.

"Look, I know all of this is way above your pay grade, and since you don't get paid as a volunteer, it's not hard to do. You are only in charge of the Red Cross nurses, not the decisions made by others. But what happened, and what may happen again, does affect the nurses you assign to work with her. I now understand why you felt helpless to do anything about this, but you do know you can expect the same thing to happen again. You have to prepare your nurses by giving them the tools to deal with McNutter the next time she manages a shelter."

Alice's voice sounded strained. "I did talk to Stan Lawrence, the head of the Regional Emergency Services Committee. I understand Jan called him and asked him to intervene, which I believe he did without hesitation."

"That's right, and thank God she did because I wouldn't have known enough to call him. I didn't even know who he was. I'm fortunate that Jan had him on her speed dial. How many of your other nurses know who he is, or what he does and have his phone number?"

"None that I know of, but I'll get his number for you, and you can call him whenever you come across a situation like this again."

"That's a start in the right direction, but we need to go further. You need to tell all of your Red Cross nurses what to do when they run into the roadblocks I did. They need to be given the chain of command, the roles of each person and their phone numbers.

"Our problem was with McNutter, but the truth is that this same situation could come up with anybody. When I ran the medical clinics in the other three shelters, it was a Red Cross staff member who was the shelter manager. When did this change?"

"When we were forced to join the regional district."

"So in many ways, we lost control over our local chapter?" I asked.

"I wouldn't go that far..."

"I would. So now I realize that we can no longer control who is put in charge of an active shelter. It could be the dogcatcher from Dorchester for all we know. In fact, I would have preferred that it was the dogcatcher instead of McNutter."

"I think that's pushing it a bit."

"I don't. We need to have a meeting with all of the Red Cross nurses. I know you can't give them the sordid details, but you can give them a few 'what ifs' and work through to the solution, which may end up being to 'Call Stan the man at the top.'"

"I'll have to check with Stan about that, but you know I'm in a difficult position and can't be specific with the nurses about who we are discussing."

"I know. One more thing. I'm not going to ever put myself in that position again, so take me off the list of nurses who will work the shelters."

"Terri, we only have about four nurses besides yourself who will take a shelter assignment."

"Do you know that the charge nurse of the Medical Services Corps gets paid for what she does? You have been volunteering in this position for over a decade. How do you have time to recruit and train nurses? It's not fair to you. What's that old saying? Put your money where your mouth is?

"If the Red Cross wants to be visible to nurses and bring them into the organization, they need to pay you to do what's necessary to recruit more nurses. If something doesn't change, the MRC will be taking over positions the Red Cross nurses once held."

"I have to go. Thanks for discussing this with me." She hung up.

I stood staring at the phone for a few minutes and then pulled a piece of paper out of my pocket and unfolded it. I dialed the number on the paper.

"Hello, Jan? It's Terri. Remember your offer to have me volunteer for the Medical Reserve Corps?"

"Yes, of course. Why?"

"When do I start?"

Chapter 23
POSTLUDE

March 7, 2013

Cape Cod Times,
March 7, 2013

Regional emergency planners are vowing not to be caught off guard again after finding themselves short on volunteers and facing criticism

Shelter chiefs weather storm

Critics blast planners for failing to open all 6 emergency facilities during the Feb. 8 blizzard.

over a decision not to open all of Cape Cod's regional shelters during the February blizzard and hurricane. A local shelter had to be opened when the generator failed in one of the regional shelters. The building's generator and floor plan were determined not to be ideal for weathering this storm. Officials are looking for an alternative to using this shelter for future storms.

Regional emergency planners "dropped the ball" by voting not to open all of the shelters, said Stan Lawrence, the head of the Cape's Coalition of Emergency Services. "Previous storms in which few people used the shelters lulled us into complacency. In the future these decisions will be dictated by projected weather conditions, not by vote. We are taking the vote out of the planning process. When all is said and done, sheltering our citizens is not the responsibility of the Red Cross or the Medical Reserve Corps. It is the responsibility of the Coalition of Emergency Services."

Lawrence gave the volunteers high praise for their hard work during this massive storm. He praised the volunteers who worked under dire circumstances in the Shelton shelter when the back-up generator failed during a power outage. He added that he will take a second look at who is chosen to manage the shelters during the storms so that they will be fully prepared for this assignment. He plans that in the future, all shelter managers will be required to attend a training program and understand all the protocols

Epilogue

A lot has changed since that massive storm, called Nemo, left residents without electricity and running water for weeks and plunged the Shelton shelter into darkness in the middle of the night. Since then, emergency planning has improved and a regionalized shelter system allows for better judgment in the management of those shelters.

Towns are no longer on their own to provide shelter managers. The regional sheltering program has a central communications system run by satellite. Emergency officials now are in direct contact with each other, holding conference calls with municipal and public safety representatives from every Cape town, as well as people from the National Grid, Comcast, Verizon, and OpenCape Corp.

Each shelter must now have a functioning generator and a ham radio in operation. Emergency management experts have upgraded their weather forecasting with a Doppler radar system to provide more timely alerts and tracking.

I've had people tell me what I "should have done." I "should have" arranged on my own for an ambulance to remove the patients at risk. I "should have" called the police or EMTs on my own. Maybe they were right or maybe they just had to be there to understand the situation.

Nurses tend to blame themselves for any failures that affect their patients. We are all rescuers. It's a trait that is often referred to as the "White Knight Syndrome." I always think that there is one more thing that I can do to make my patients better or at least more comfortable. It's a flaw, I know, because we can't always make people better but we struggle to try and when we fail, we take it as a personal failure.

We question ourselves. Is our judgment wrong? Are we too weak to deal with the tough situations that face us? At the end of the shift, we often leave our places of work mulling about what else we "should" have or "could" have done.

I'm grateful to the nurse from the Medical Reserve Corps who shared this experience with me and successfully found a way out of unforeseen circumstances, mounting surprises, and erratic managers. She knew what we needed to do to get our patients the help they needed and was daring enough to do it.

I like to think that the flaws found with the Shelton shelter have paved the way for improved services going forward. I believe it was a lesson learned from the past for the entire emergency system and provided a basis for better planning and management.

I can also find some solace knowing that with those improvements, no nurse in charge of the medical services in these shelters will ever have to experience what I did, and that in itself, is enough to make me proud.

APPENDIX

SAFETY TIPS FROM THE AMERICAN RED CROSS

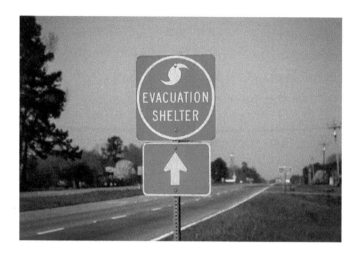

10 Things to Bring to a Hurricane Shelter

In the event of a hurricane, the number-one question is whether to stay in town or evacuate to a safer environment. Numerous communities offer a great resource: hurricane shelters. Each area provides a safe building for families in the community to come together and ride out the storm in a sturdy, secure setting. But a hurricane shelter may fill up fast, and supplies are limited.

Below is a list of essential items to bring with you to a hurricane shelter.

1. Medication

Make sure you have more than three days of medication with you. If it's prescription medication, you'll need to order more well before the hurricane comes. Pharmacies will most likely be closed days before or after the hurricane, depending on the amount of damage.

2. Water and Food

If you're staying in a shelter, there will be many people in your community who have sought refuge there as well. Everyone will be hungry and thirsty, so it's important to bring your own food and water to ensure that you and your family have a supply. Don't forget to take a can opener if you're bringing canned, nonperishable food.

3. Flashlight and Weather Radio

Having a weather radio is important because it keeps you updated on weather conditions. There's also a good chance that the electricity will go out during the storm, so take a flashlight with you to have a reliable light source and extra batteries.

4. Clothing

A comfortable change of clothing is essential. There's no telling how long the hurricane will last, or when it will be safe to leave the shelter. Wear and bring clothes that are comfy and easy to wear.

5. Bedding

It's important to bring blankets, sleeping bags, pillows, and other comfortable items for sitting and sleeping. Although a shelter may offer blankets and pillows, it's better to be on the safe side and have your own with you.

6. Entertainment Items

Toys, books, and other non-electric items are vital. You'll be in a shelter with most likely no electricity and plenty of time to fill. In order to stay occupied with some entertainment, bring board games, cards, puzzles, or any other activity you enjoy.

7. First Aid Supplies
Bring a first aid kit in case of an emergency. After the storm, there may be dangerous debris around the hurricane shelter and someone could get injured.

8. Hygiene
Bring a toothbrush, toothpaste, soap, deodorant, and any other personal hygiene products you regularly use.

9. Personal Information
Store your important personal information in a waterproof bag. This includes Social Security cards, birth certificates, and medical records, as well as other valuable documents.

10. Cash
It will be important to have some cash with you, especially after the hurricane. Just like pharmacies, banks will most likely be out of service. Electricity may also be down, so credit or debit cards will be of no use.

POWER FAILURE

FOLLOW THESE SAFETY STEPS AS WINTER STORMS HIT YOUR COMMUNITY

As dangerous winter weather continues to plague most of the country, the American Red Cross urges everyone to stay safe and stay at home if possible, and offers these steps to follow:

GET RED CROSS READY

Make sure you have enough heating fuel on hand. Stay indoors and wear warm clothes. Layers of loose-fitting, lightweight, warm clothing will keep you warmer than a bulky sweater. Check on relatives, neighbors and friends, particularly if they are elderly or if they live alone. Keep your vehicle's gas tank full to keep the fuel line from freezing.

Don't forget your pets. Bring your companion animals indoors. Create a place where your other animals can be comfortable in severe winter weather.

GENERATOR SAFETY

If you are using a generator, keep it dry and don't use it in wet conditions.

- Never use a generator, grill, camp stove or other gasoline, propane, natural gas or charcoal-burning devices inside a home, garage, basement, crawlspace, or any partially enclosed area. Keep these devices outside away from doors, windows and vents, which could allow carbon monoxide to come indoors.
- Operate the generator on a dry surface under an open canopy-like structure, such as under a tarp held up by poles.
- Don't touch a generator with wet hands.
- Turn the generator off and let it cool down before refueling. Gasoline spilled on hot engine parts could ignite.
- Plug appliances directly into the generator. Never try to power the house wiring by plugging the generator into a wall outlet.

IF THE POWER IS OUT

- Use flashlights in the dark — not candles.

- If you must go out during a winter storm, use public transportation if possible. Eliminate unnecessary travel, especially by car. Traffic lights will be out and roads will be congested.

- Turn off and unplug all unnecessary electrical equipment.

- Turn off or disconnect any appliances and electronics that you were using when the power went out. When power comes back on, surges or spikes can damage equipment.

- Leave one light on, so you'll know when power is restored.

- During a prolonged outage, keep refrigerator and freezer doors closed as much as possible to protect your food.

- First, use perishable food from the refrigerator. Perishables are safe to eat when they have a temperature of 40 degrees Fahrenheit or below. Then, use food from the freezer.

- If the power outage will continue beyond a day, prepare a cooler with ice for your freezer items. Keep food in a dry, cool spot and cover it at all times.

STAY SAFE OUTSIDE

- Wear layered clothing, mittens or gloves, and a hat. Outer garments should be tightly woven and water repellent.

- Cover your mouth to protect your lungs from severely cold air. Avoid taking deep breaths; minimize talking.

- Keep dry. Change wet clothing frequently to prevent a loss of body heat.

- Stretch before you go out. If you go out to shovel snow, do a few stretching exercises first to reduce your chances of muscle injury.

- Avoid overexertion, such as shoveling heavy snow, pushing a vehicle, or walking in deep snow. The strain may cause a heart attack. Sweating could lead to a chill and hypothermia.

- Walk carefully on snowy, icy sidewalks. Slips and falls occur frequently in winter weather, resulting in painful and some-times disabling injuries.

- Get out of the cold immediately if the signs of hypothermia and frostbite appear.

- Signs of frostbite include lack of feeling in the affected area or skin that appears waxy, is cold to the touch, or is discolored (flushed, white or gray, yellow or blue)

WHAT TO DO FOR FROSTBITE:

- Move the person to a warm place
- Handle the area gently; never rub the affected area
- Warm gently by soaking the affected area in warm water (100–105 degrees F) until it appears red and feels warm
- Loosely bandage the area with dry, sterile dressings
- If the person's fingers or toes are frostbitten, place dry, sterile gauze between them to keep them separated
- Avoid breaking any blisters
- Do not allow the affected area to refreeze
- Seek professional medical care as soon as possible

Signs of hypothermia include shivering, numbness or weakness, a glassy stare, apathy or impaired judgment or loss of consciousness.

WHAT TO DO FOR HYPOTHERMIA:
- CALL 9-1-1 or the local emergency number
- Gently move the person to a warm place
- Monitor breathing and circulation
- Give rescue breathing and CPR if needed
- Remove any wet clothing and dry the person
- Warm the person slowly by wrapping in blankets or by putting dry clothing on the person.
- Hot water bottles and chemical hot packs may be used when first wrapped in a towel or blanket before applying. Do not warm the person too quickly, such as by immersing him or her in warm water.
- Warm the core first (trunk, abdomen), not the extremities (hands, feet).

PREVENT FROZEN PIPES

- Keep garage doors closed if there are water supply lines in the garage.

- Open kitchen and bathroom cabinet doors to allow warmer air to circulate around the plumbing.

- Let the cold water drip from the faucet served by exposed pipes. Running water through the pipe - even at a trickle - helps prevent pipes from freezing.

- Keep the thermostat set to the same temperature both during the day and at night.

- If you will be going away during cold weather, leave the heat on in your home, set to a temperature no lower than 55° F.

HOW TO THAW FROZEN PIPES

- If you turn on a faucet and only a trickle comes out, suspect a frozen pipe. Likely places for frozen pipes include against exterior walls or where your water service enters your home through the foundation.

- Keep the faucet open. As you treat the frozen pipe and the frozen area begins to melt, water will begin to flow through the frozen area. Running water through the pipe will help melt ice in the pipe.

- Apply heat to the section of pipe using an electric heating pad wrapped around the pipe, an electric hair dryer, a portable space heater (kept away from flammable materials), or by wrapping pipes with towels soaked in hot water. Do not use a blowtorch, kerosene or propane heater, charcoal stove, or other open flame device.

- Apply heat until full water pressure is restored. If you are unable to locate the frozen area, if the frozen area is not accessible, or if you cannot thaw the pipe, call a licensed plumber.

- Check all other faucets in your home to find out if you have additional frozen pipes. If one pipe freezes, others may freeze, too.

HOME HEATING SAFETY

- Keep all potential sources of fuel like paper, clothing, bedding or rugs at least three feet away from space heaters, stoves, or fireplaces.

- Don't leave portable heaters and fireplaces unattended. Turn off space heaters and make sure any embers in the fireplace are extinguished before going to bed or leaving home.

- Place space heaters on a level, hard and nonflammable surface, not on rugs or carpets or near bedding or drapes. Keep children and pets away from space heaters.

- Never use a cooking range or oven to heat your home.

- Keep fire in your fireplace by using a glass or metal fire screen large enough to catch sparks and rolling logs.

DOWNLOAD APPS

People can download the Red Cross Emergency App for instant access to weather alerts for their area and where loved ones live. Expert medical guidance and a hospital locator are included in the First Aid App in case travelers encounter any mishaps. Both apps are available to download for free in app stores or at redcross.org/apps.

ABOUT THE AMERICAN RED CROSS:

The American Red Cross shelters, feeds, and provides emotional support to victims of disasters; supplies about 40 percent of the nation's blood; teaches skills that save lives; provides international humanitarian aid; and supports military members and their families. The Red Cross is a not-for-profit organization that depends on volunteers and the generosity of the American public to perform its mission. For more information, please visit redcross.org or cruzrojaamericana.org, or visit us on Twitter at @RedCross.

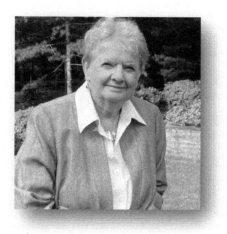

ABOUT THE AUTHOR

Terri Arthur, RN, BS, MS is a former volunteer disaster nurse for the American Red Cross and a charter member of the Nightingale Society in recognition for her generous support for nursing scholarship and research. For her work advocating for the health and safety of nurses, she was awarded the Kathryn McGinn-Cutler Award from the Massachusetts Nurses Association.

Arthur's book, *Fatal Decision: Edith Cavell, WWI Nurse*, won the Midwest Independent Publishers Award for Historical Fiction and was also a finalist for the Eric Hoffer Award, an international competition.

It was also awarded the Boston Massachusetts State House Citation of Recognition. The story has been optioned for film.

She is a former adjunct professor for Lesley University Graduate School, Cambridge, Massachusetts, and the former nursing director of SEAK, a company that provides continuing education to nurses, doctors, and lawyers on occupational health and safety.

In addition to being an author, Terri has worked as a critical care nurse, staff educator, and clinical manager. She holds degrees in nursing, education, and biology and a master's degree in health business management. She founded and continues to manage Medical Education Systems, Inc., an educational company.

Terri's writings have been published in the *Journal of Emergency Nursing*, *The American Nurses Association Online Journal of Issues in Nursing*, the *Navy Medical Magazine of History*, the *Nursing Standard* in England, the American Red Cross on-line magazine *Nursing Matters Past and Present*, the *American Association for the History of Nursing*, and many other newspapers and magazines.

She is a frequently requested guest lecturer nationally and internationally speaking to historical societies, colleges, nursing schools, hospitals, women's groups, military groups, and nursing associations.

Contact information via her website:
www.TerriArthur.com

Email: terri.arthur@gmail.com